The Autophagy Diet

Remove Toxicity and Provide Energy to Obtain A Rapid Weight Loss and Anti-Aging Process Through Ketogenic Diet, Intermittent Fasting and Extended Water

By Agatha Franklin

Table of Contents

Chapter 1: What is Autophagy?

Autophagy is a natural process that occurs in our body at a cellular level. It involves breaking down old, damaged cells and reusing them for fuel. Proteins and other materials contained in the destroyed cell matter are used to form new, stronger, and healthier cells. This is a fascinating event because it literally cleans up cell waste that would otherwise remain stored in our body. In simple terms, autophagy rejuvenates our body and provides many benefits as a result. Although autophagy has become a buzzword and an interesting topic of discussion among diet experts and professionals, it is far from being a new concept. The autophagy process begins at a point when our body requires fuel for building and repairing new cells and tissues. On a cellular scale, we use the nutrients and energy from the food we consume, usually in the form of glucose. When we consume a diet low in carbs, such as the ketogenic diet, we use up the glucose quickly, which is converted from the carbohydrates and switch to burning fat stores. Once we use all that we have, our body will continue to search for materials to break down and use. This is when autophagy takes effect: our body will identify old, damaged cellular waste and use it for energy.

In ancient societies, our ancestors benefitted from autophagy during long periods of fasting and eating whole foods low in carbohydrates and sugars, such as a wild game, berries and leafy greens, all of which could be hunted and gathered. Processed foods were not available, and our ancestors were more physically active, as this was the only means to obtain food. Periods of fasting would occur in between meals, as food could not be adequately stored as today, in refrigerators and freezers. Just over a century ago, people consumed more wholesome foods, as a ready-made, packaged meals only became popular once life became busier in the 1950s, leaving less time to prepare and enjoy foods in their natural state.

Thousands of years ago, when there was no food available for longer periods of time, people simply did not eat and had to search and seek out food sources available, in the form of foraging through forests and jungles to hunting. During these periods, people would naturally fast or abstain from food, which has benefits on its own and leads to the onset of autophagy, which is explained further in chapter ___. A clearer mind, and better focus and clarity, were considered among the benefits of fasting, as the food was a distraction. Fasting was also practiced in ancient times for other reasons as well, including for religious practices and spiritual reasons. During food shortage, or in between hunting and harvesting, fasting was a regular occurrence and circumstantial. Fasting can last from several hours during a 24-hour period to several days. It is currently practiced by many people in the form of intermittent fasting, which refers to extended periods of time between meals, though not necessarily for more than a day at a time.

The Autophagy Process

The basic science of how autophagy works to "clean" our bodies and rejuvenate cells. The word autophagy literally translates as "self-eating" or self-consuming. It is our body's way of developing a recycling program, making our bodies more efficient at identifying faulty or broken parts, including cancerous cells, and other materials that can cause or contribute to harm, such as obesity and chronic metabolic issues. The science behind autophagy is fascinating, and research is ongoing to determine the risks and benefits of its powerful effects. Also known as autophagocytosis, this occurs when proteins inside of the double-membrane vesicle inside cells, which are extracted and moved into the lysosome. Lysosomes are surrounded by a membrane, and also contain hydrolytic enzymes that work together to break down proteins, nucleic acids and other materials found in cells that can be recycled and reused in the building of new cells and tissues. Studies conducted in laboratories indicate that a significant reduction in caloric intake, and more specifically, fasting, will trigger this process.

The results of this research indicate a decline in certain conditions in rats and mice, such as weight loss, increased longevity, and metabolism occurred after just twenty-four hours of fasting. At this time, high levels of autophagosomes were found in their bodies, indicating a state of autophagy.

During the autophagy process, two main hormones become involved: glucagon and insulin. As insulin levels rise, the level of glucagon decreases, and the same occurs in reverse: when glucagon increases, insulin falls. When glucagon rises, it stimulates the production of autophagosomes, and autophagy begins. The approximate time frame for inducing this process is a fast of approximately fifteen hours. This gives your body enough time to reduce insulin, though a longer fast means better results, which is usually closer to a full twenty-four hours. The role diet plays in our daily lives and how we schedule our meals has a significant impact on how we can benefit from autophagy and determining when it will work best to maximize its potential.

Chapter 2: How Does Autophagy Play a Role in Diet?

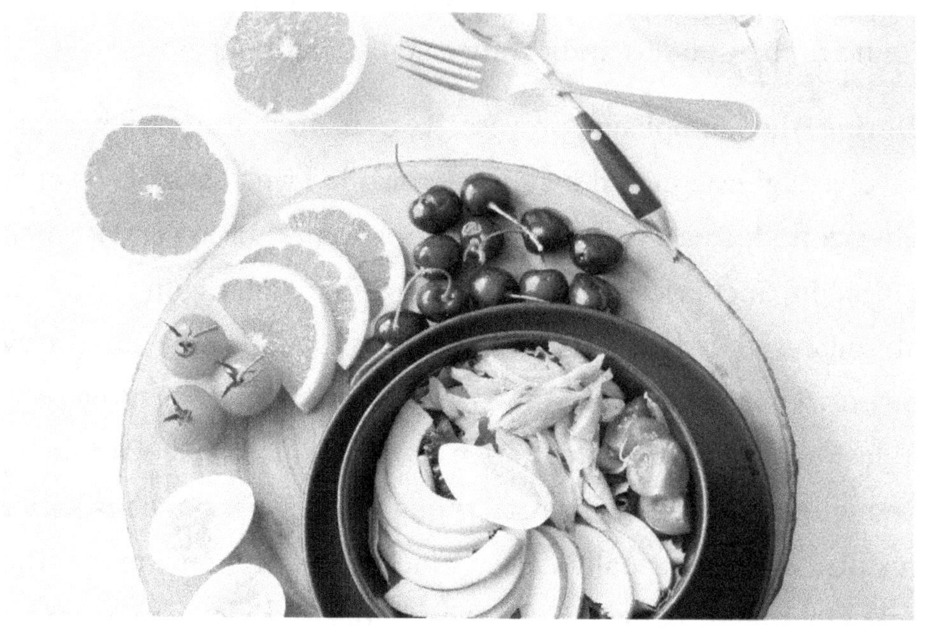

Autophagy plays a major role in our diet in several ways: what we eat and when we eat. These two factors, the what and when determine how quickly we can shift into a state of autophagy, and during which time frame within that window of opportunity is the most efficient and beneficial to reap the rewards of this cellular clean up process. To begin this process, it's best to prepare and plan ahead carefully and avoid "jumping" into an all-or-nothing approach, such as a 24-hour fast without any preparation or prior fasting experience or eliminating all high carb foods overnight with little to no options for replacement. One of the most important factors of the autophagy diet, as with any diet that is expected to make significant results, is to plan, prepare, and take time to adjust in stages. For example, going from a standard way of eating, which often includes a lot of sugars and carbohydrates, to a low carb, whole food diet with periods of intermittent fasting is a major shift, and your body will react accordingly. For this reason, it's best to begin the change in the diet gradually at a level that works best for you and your body.

How to Begin an Autophagy Diet

Beginning the autophagy diet is more of a process than a meal plan. This includes implementing several new ways of approaching diet and food planning to achieve a state of autophagy, by reducing the body's reliance on carbohydrates as the main fuel source and moving towards becoming fat adapted. During this phase, on a cellular level, your body will benefit from periods of fasting, which can occur in smaller time frames on a daily basis, or for longer periods of a day or more. Once your body is burning fat for fuel, shifting into fasting will take you towards achieving autophagy, where your body has used up its fuel sources and begins to search for the old, damaged cellular matter to use as energy.

To begin the journey to autophagy, consider the plan in stages, by first implementing either an intermittent fasting schedule or a low carb diet, both of which will limit your carb and calorie intake. Once you become comfortable with either the fasting schedule or diet, you can implement both, alternating between regular eating of low carb (preferably ketogenic) foods and periods of fasting.

Chapter 3: Why Choose Autophagy? The Benefits and Risks of this Diet

Are there risks as well as benefits to this diet? Can autophagy cause problems along with the positive results? The effects of autophagy are phenomenal and fascinating for many people, though there are also side effects and risks associated with intermittent fasting, low carb eating combined to reach this state. It is also not always a good choice for some people while remaining a significant benefit to others, for the following reasons:

- If you have an eating disorder of already established bad eating habits, such as skipping meals frequently, for this reason, intermittent fasting is not a good choice. The difference between fasting in between meals and skipping them is the planned and calculated approach, which is used in the fasting process, whereas skipping meals with little or no planning can be harmful, particularly if you don't eat the right foods or very small amounts in between skipping them. For intermittent fasting to work effectively, and lead to autophagy, a good, healthy way of eating should be established before moving into a fasting state, so that your body has enough nutrients available.

- If you have type 1 diabetes, it's important to maintain consistent insulin levels, which may be a challenge during intermittent fasting and a ketogenic diet. If you have this condition and are seriously considering an autophagy diet plan, it's best to consult a doctor first. Alternatively, progressing to a state of autophagy through intermittent fasting and low carb foods can prevent type 2 diabetes and control its progression in cases where it has already started. The difference between type 1 and 2 diabetes: type 1 is when the body doesn't produce enough or any insulin at all, and type 2 can vary from maintaining high insulin to not enough. Type 1 diabetes must be carefully monitored medically and requires regular doses of insulin, whereas the type 2 condition can be controlled and treated through a healthy diet, which is how low carb eating and fasting can be beneficial

- Intermittent fasting is not advised for women who are pregnant or breastfeeding. It's also best to avoid while trying to conceive. Low carb and ketogenic diets are best postpartum, instead of during pregnancy or breastfeeding, as our bodies need the extra fuel for energy.

- Anyone under the age of 18 should avoid the goal of autophagy altogether. As you grow and develop, it's vital not to limit caloric intake or carbohydrates, unless under the supervision of a doctor for medical reasons. It is a goal best suited for adults for the purpose of improving health and losing weight. For older adults, autophagy is an ideal option to slow down the aging process, the benefits of which are covered in this book.

Overall, autophagy is a process that shouldn't be considered lightly and may take a while to work towards. The steps that lead to autophagy, intermittent, and long-term fasting, as well as ketogenic or low carb dieting, can take a while to adjust to if they are new concepts. Each step is a journey in itself, to explore and try different approaches, until you feel comfortable enough to progress further, with the ultimate goal of reaching autophagy.

Chapter 4: The Different Ways to Approach an Autophagy Diet

There are several paths to achieve autophagy, all of which reduce the caloric intake of foods, thereby reducing insulin and increasing the body's ability to shift into ketosis, which leads to producing autophagosomes. There are individual factors to consider, including the level of physical activity, current eating habits, and diet. Aside from achieving autophagy, there are beneficial ways to eat and fast that can support an easier shift to cellular rejuvenation, and an overall improvement in how your body feels and functions.

Extended water fasts

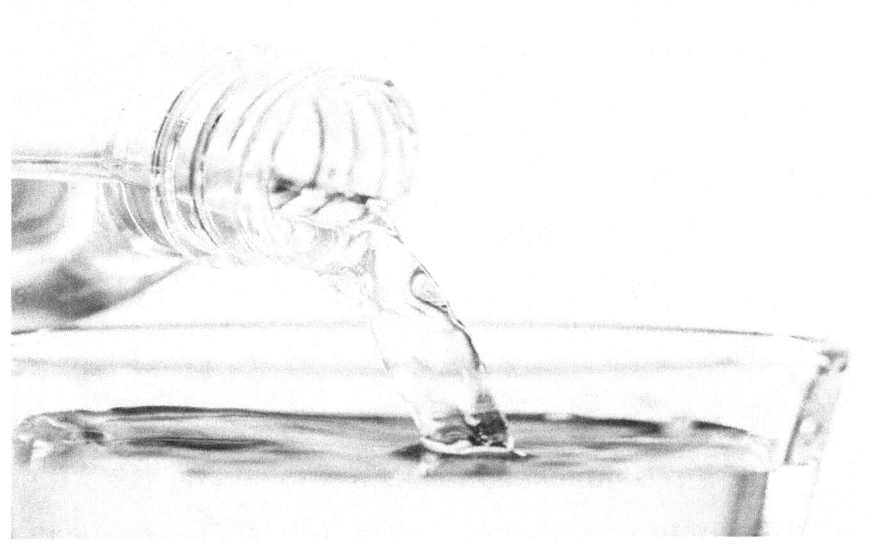

Fasting, more specifically, intermittent fasting, is one of the most effective methods of weight loss and encouraging autophagy. Water fasting essentially involves fasting for short or intermediate periods of time, while drinking lots of water to remain hydrated and flush toxins. This method of fasting restricts all foods and drinks, except water, for the duration of the fast. A water fast is beneficial for several reasons:

- It keeps hunger from developing. Water is often what we need when we experience hunger, which is one of the first signs of dehydration or thirst. Drinking water regularly, especially during a fast, reduces these false hunger pangs

- Even during short periods of water fasting, research indicates a reduction in blood pressure, cholesterol and heart disease, better metabolism, and weight loss.

- Improved concentration and energy. If your fast includes water that is filtered and re-mineralized (minerals are added back after removal with other elements), you'll continue to have the benefits of these nutrients while you abstain from food.

- Water fasting can be done easily from 24 hours for up to 3 days. It is recommended to begin with shorter periods of fasting, from 16 to 18 hours, prior to extending to one full day or more.

- Without the inclusion of carbohydrates during this fast, your body will use fat stores to burn for fuel and energy, which increases the potential for weight loss

Ketogenic Diet and the Basics of Ketosis

The ketogenic diet is a way of eating that centers around increasing the healthy fats while strictly reducing carbohydrates to less than (or up to) 20 grams per day. This diet was developed around the 1930s to treat many health conditions, such as seizures resulting from epilepsy, insulin regulation, and other diseases and conditions difficult to treat with conventional therapy. Reducing the carbohydrates significantly was the key to success for the treatments of these and many other conditions. Studies conducted in more recent years indicate numerous benefits, including fighting (and preventing) type 2 diabetes, brain, and cognitive function, preventing Alzheimer's and other related diseases. Weight loss and insulin regulation are two major results that have given the keto diet a significant amount of popularity recently, with many dieticians and medical professionals either supporting or criticizing the low carb way of eating.

Ketosis is a state that shifts your body's prime fuel source from carbohydrates and glucose to fats stored in the body. By reducing the number of carbs in your diet, the body will default to fat stores. During this process, the liver produces ketones, which indicates ketosis is in effect, and the body is fat adapted or in fat-burning mode. The ketones increase as the glucose falls, and the body has no other sources of energy. There are three types of ketones that result during this process:

- Acetoacetate (known as AcAc)

- 3beta-hydroxybutyrate (3HB)

- Acetone

The first two, AcAc and 3HB are the most abundant of the three, while acetone is produced during the body's expelling of ketones, and in trace amounts. The presence of ketones can be detected by test strips, which are often available at a pharmacy or drug store. Blood tests and testing the level of ketones in breath are two other methods, though test strips that detect ketones in urine are most popular and most accurate. While testing for ketones is not a requirement of the diet, it is often done to confirm the onset of ketosis and track its progress over a duration of time. The following scale is used to determine the level of ketosis, based on the production of ketones:

No ketosis	Trace amount	More than a trace, close to a small amount	Moderate or medium amount	Significant amount	Large/excessive amount
0	0.5	1.5	3.5-4.0	4.0 and higher	8.0

According to research on the correlation between ketosis and weight loss, the ideal spot for losing weight is between 1.5-3.0. These figures represent the presence of ketones in the blood in mmol/L. Between 15-622 mg/dL is the preferred or recommended range for weight loss. While ketosis is beneficial for weight loss, especially if this state is reached and maintained for a length of time, moving into a state of autophagy may require a longer period of time, with intermittent fasting included, in order to exhaust the glucose in the body.

Intermittent Fasting

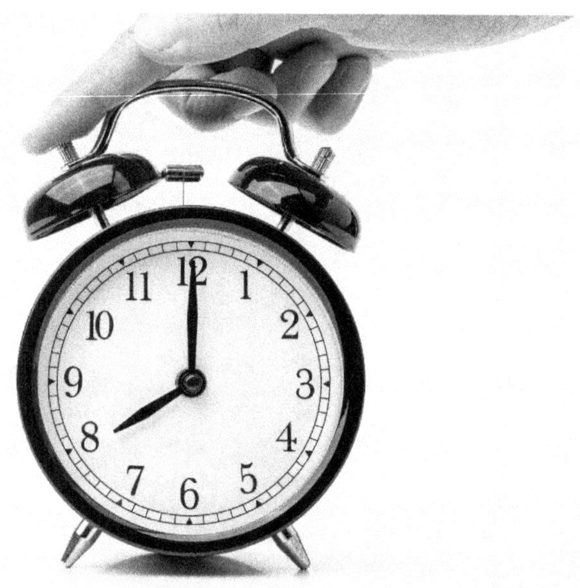

Intermittent fasting is becoming increasingly more common as studies show a lot of benefits from short-term fasts in between cycles of regular eating. When most people consider fasting, long-term avoidance of food and water for long periods of time, even days, may come to mind. While long-term fasting, for 24 hours or more, can be very beneficial, it is not recommended for everyone and should be a goal worked towards on a gradual, careful basis by trying shorter periods of time. While intermittent fasting denotes smaller periods of time, there are variations in the number of hours allocated between fasting, and feasting. For example, in a typical day, we may eat from 7:00 am, starting with breakfast, followed by lunch, a snack and dinner around 6 or 7 pm, our window would effectively be 12 hours, from 7 to 7, otherwise known as 12:12. The 12:12 refers to a 12-hour window to eat and the remaining 12 hours is fasting, for a total of one day, or 24 hours.

The Basics of Fasting

During a fast, drinking water is permitted, as well as any liquid that will not increase the glucose levels in your body. Acceptable options include water, tea, and coffee (with no sugar, sweeteners, milk or other additives), and sparkling or carbonated water. There are some carbonated beverages that have low or no-carb sweeteners, which may be included in moderate amounts, as they will not have an impact on the fasting process. Bone broth is sometimes consumed during a fast, though the opinions vary on whether this is recommended. Some experts will advise against it, as bone broth contains minerals and ingredients that essentially "break" a fast, though others recommend it as a way to continually get nutrients while enjoying all the benefits of a fast. The variance in opinion hinges on whether adding the broth is significant enough to impede the progress of fasting, or if it may enhance its potential.

For the purposes of autophagy, consuming anything, including water during a fast, can slow down the progression towards the production of autophagosomes, even if slightly. For this reason, it's often suggested to minimize water and liquids, or simply "dry" fast, which refers to avoiding all foods and drinks. Why do small or moderate amounts of liquids slow down the onset of autophagy? This is because our bodies will use anything that becomes available to use for repairing and building new cells and tissues, including the properties of water. While this is a small amount, and will not stop autophagy from occurring, especially during longer fasting periods, avoidance of all liquids is an option to clear the path towards achieving autophagy much sooner.

Different Types of Fasting

Each plan for intermittent fasting is divided into "windows" to identify when eating is permitted or when it is abstained from. A "fasting" window indicates fasting is in progress, and no food or drink is consumed. There are some exceptions that may be considered, which will be covered in this section, following the fasting methods. During the eating of feeding "window," food and drink are permitted as per your own way of eating, whether there are no changes made at all, or a new diet is started, such as ketogenic or low-calorie plan. If you decide to make significant changes to your diet, in conjunction with intermittent fasting, it's best to begin one plan first to get accustomed to it, before adding more changes. For example, begin eating low carb foods and reducing the overall carbohydrates and sugar in our diet, prior to adding periods of fasting. Alternatively, you can begin adjusting your schedule to intermittent fasting windows, gradually increasing the fasting window until you find a plan that works best, followed by changing your diet within each eating window.

The most advantageous aspect of intermittent fasting, which focus on when to eat, rather than what to eat, is the way it can be individualized to fit within your schedule for work, eating and rest. Although intermittent fasting does not specify which types of foods or diet to eat, adapting to and maintaining a low carb diet with wholesome foods is strongly recommended for best results. Combining the ketogenic diet with intermittent fasting, for example, while not a requirement, is often done to maximize the results of both ways of eating. This plan may also bring about autophagy more quickly than intermittent fasting without low carb eating, as glucose is already significantly reduced during eating hours. The following types of intermittent fasting plans are recommended in the following order:

12:12 Fasting Method: For Beginners

This is the easiest intermittent fasting plan, to begin with, as it will "train" or adapt your body and mind to the idea of timing your meals and eating within a specified window of hours or timeframe. The 12:12 method is realistic for people with no prior experience, as it is compatible with most regular daily eating schedules and eating routines. Planning this starter-fast option is as easy as choosing when to begin and stop each fasting and eating window:

<u>12:12 Plan A:</u>

This fasting plan begins on a Sunday evening after 7 pm, with the fasting "window" or period during which there is no food or drink, and ending the following morning at 7 am, when breakfast is served.

Day of the week	Sunday	Monday	Tuesday	Wednesday	Thursday	Friday	Saturday
Feeding or eating window	7 am to 7 pm (dinner is between 6-7 pm)	7 am to 7 pm	7 am to 7 pm	7 am to 7 pm	7 am to 7 pm	7 am to 7 pm	7 am to 7 pm
Fasting	7 pm to 7	7 pm to 7	7 pm to 7	7 pm to 7	7 pm to 7	7 pm to 7	7 pm to 7

| windo w | am the next morni ng | am the next mor ning | am the next mor ning | am the next morni ng | am the next morn ing | am the next mor ning | am the next mor ning |

This plan provides a generous window of eating between the daytime hours of 7 am to 7 pm, allowing more than enough time to enjoy breakfast, lunch, and dinner with periods of drinking and/or snacks in between. When fasting begins after 7 pm, no eating will occur until breakfast the following day, which begins at 7 am or later. The fasting hours or "window" can include sleeping, and usually does, as it makes the plan easier to follow and most people would not eat during the night. Another option for this plan, depending on your individual schedule, may look like plan B:

12:12 Plan B:

Day of the week	Sunda y	Mon day	Tues day	Wedne sday	Thur sday	Frid ay	Satur day
Feedin g or eating windo	5am to 5pm (dinne r is	5am to 5pm	5am to 5pm	5am to 5pm	5am to 5pm	5am to 5pm	5am to 5pm

w	betwe en 4-5 pm or skippe d altoget her)						
Fastin g windo w	5pm to 5am the next morni ng	5pm to 5am the next mor ning	5pm to 5am the next mor ning	5pm to 5am the next morni ng	5pm to 5am the next morn ing	5pm to 5am the next mor ning	5pm to 5am the next mor ning

The second plan, which includes a fasting window of 5pm to 5am, is best suited to someone with an early start, providing a better opportunity to fit more meals earlier into the day while starting the fast at 5pm. This shift in hours, compared to the 7 to 7 plans in plan A, is a good fit for a meal plan that includes a large breakfast and lunch, with the option for a snack, and either no dinner or a light meal just prior to 5pm. The third option (below) is a good option for beginning the eating window later in the day if it is preferred to skip or delay breakfast for a brunch or early lunch.

<u>12:12 Plan C:</u>

Day of the week	Sunday	Monday	Tuesday	Wednesday	Thursday	Friday	Saturday
Feeding or eating window	12 pm to 12am (breakfast is either skipped or shifted later or as an early lunch)	12 pm to 12am	12 pm to 12am	12 pm to 12am	12 pm to 12am	12 pm to 12am	12 pm to 12am
Fasting window	12am to 12 pm the following day	12am to 12 pm the following day	12am to 12 pm the following day	12am to 12 pm the following day	12am to 12 pm the following day	12am to 12 pm the following day	12am to 12 pm the following day

The later fasting window beginning at 12 pm until 12am provides later options for meals and works well for people who do not wish to include breakfast in their daily plan, and instead, shift their lunch and dinner meals later, leaving an option for a later snack before 12am. This plan also works well for people who work and/or go to bed late.

The 12:12 intermittent fasting plan will not get you into ketosis, nor will it accomplish a state of autophagy, unless food during the eating window is severely restricted, which is not recommended until you are ready for a longer fast, which will bring about both ketosis and autophagy. The benefits of this method lie in the following principles, which are established during the beginning of this plan for further success:

- Establishing a routine. If you haven't planned your meals before, intermittent fasting will give you definite time limits, so that you learn to work within these windows and budget your meals accordingly. While there is flexibility within each eating window, your meals are restricted within these hours.

- Individualizing your plan. If you have a busy schedule, planning your eating and fasting windows should be done with careful consideration of when you normally eat and/or when you desire to take your meals. Your schedule doesn't need to be etched in stone or planned for months in advance; you can shift your eating and fasting hours on a weekly or bi-weekly basis if it suits your schedule for work and other priorities.

- There are no dietary restrictions during intermittent fasting unless you choose to implement them, or otherwise already restrict certain foods, calories or carbs in your diet. The focus is on when to eat and expanding the fasting window will automatically keep your caloric intake and total carbs lower during the fasting hours.

Once you have adapted to a 12:12 diet, the next step is to expand the fasting window and reducing the time frame for meals. The 16:8 is recommended for this option.

16:8 Intermittent Fasting Plan

The 16:8 method refers to an intermittent fasting schedule of 16 hours fasting and 8 hours of eating. While sixteen hours may seem like a long period of time, it is a good start for beginners, or the next step after adjusting to a 12:12 fasting plan. The 16:8 plan allows for a 16-hour fasting window, followed by an 8-hour eating window. Eating within 8 hours may seem like a far cry from 12 hours, though with a few minor adjustments, it is easy to adjust to within one or two weeks. Adjusting your meals from a 12-hour window to an 8-hour window can be as simple as shifting the same meals closer together or reducing the size and/or amount of meals. For example, if you skip a meal to fit your eating plan into a smaller time frame, add an extra light snack or simply reduce one or more of the meals, so they can be enjoyed closer together.

What does a 16:8 intermittent fasting plan look like? It can vary considerably, depending on your schedule. Like the 12:12 plan, you can begin early in the day, or later, to reflect when you wish to begin the eating window.

<u>16:8 Plan A:</u>

This fasting plan begins on a Sunday evening after 3 pm, with the fasting "window" or time period during which there is no food or drink, and ending the following morning at 7 am, when breakfast is served.

Day of the week	Sunday	Monday	Tuesday	Wednesday	Thursday	Friday	Saturday
Feeding or eating window	7 am to 3 pm (skip dinner or have a	7 am to 3 pm	7 am to 3 pm	7 am to 3 pm	7 am to 3 pm	7 am to 3 pm	7 am to 3 pm

	light snack)						
Fasting window	3 pm to 7 am the next morning	3 pm to 7 am the next morning	3 pm to 7 am the next morning	3 pm to 7 am the next morning	3 pm to 7 am the next morning	3 pm to 7 am the next morning	3 pm to 7 am the next morning

This fasting plan can work with three traditional meals: breakfast between 7-8 am, lunch at 11:30-12:30 and a light dinner or snack between 2-3 pm. Dinner can be omitted in place of a snack, or skipped altogether, if lunch is shifted to a later time, and a snack added between breakfast and lunch (mid-morning). If you tend to eat lighter meals, the 16:8 plan allows for as many as possible within the 8-hour eating window, as no food is taken during the fast.

<u>16:8 Plan B:</u>

This schedule is a variation on the 16:8 plan, which allows for a more substantial lunch and dinner, with a skipped breakfast for meal replacement in the late morning. Beginning the fasting window later in the date is an appropriate option for people who tend to skip breakfast as a habit, or prefer it later, mid-morning or skip directly to lunch for the first meal. If you have a large dinner the evening before, this can provide more sustenance until the next late morning or lunch hour.

Day of the week	Sunday	Monday	Tuesday	Wednesday	Thursday	Friday	Saturday
Feeding or eating window	11 am to 7 pm (skip breakfast or have late morning)	11 am to 7 pm	11 am to 7 pm	11 am to 7 pm	11 am to 7 pm	11 am to 7 pm	11 am to 7 pm
Fasting window	7 pm to 11 am the next morning	7 pm to 11 am the next morning	7 pm to 11 am the next morning	7 pm to 11 am the next morning	7 pm to 11 am the next morning	7 pm to 11 am the next morning	7 pm to 11 am the next morning

The 8-hour eating window resembles a standard working day or shift, which is usually between 7.5 to 8 hours each day. If you plan your eating hours just before and after work, and one or two opportunities in between, it leaves the remainder of the 24 hours as a fasting period. If you work, attend a school or other activities for an 8-hour period, the measuring process is easy and can be matched to either coincide with or overlap your eating window. If you have the type of employment that doesn't provide a lot of time to take breaks or eat, you may want to shift the hours earlier or later to accommodate.

16:8 Plan C:

In keeping with the 8-hour fasting window, the hours can be easily moved to start later, skipping breakfast with the option of moving lunch later as well, and focusing on eating later in the day, which results in breaking the fast later the following morning. This plan is ideal for people who generally start later in the day or wish to begin their eating window later. It allows for a late lunch and dinner, with a snack option in between:

Day of the week	Sunday	Monday	Tuesday	Wednesday	Thursday	Friday	Saturday
Feeding or eating	1 pm to 9 pm	1 pm to 9 pm	1 pm to 9 pm	1 pm to 9 pm	1 pm to 9 pm	1 pm to 9 pm	1 pm to 9 pm

windo w	(skip breakf ast and shift lunch and dinner later)						
Fastin g windo w	9 pm to 1 pm the next day	9 pm to 1 pm the next day	9 pm to 1 pm the next day	9 pm to 1 pm the next day	9 pm to 1 pm the next day	9 pm to 1 pm the next day	9 pm to 1 pm the next day

Aside from the suggested windows for eating and fasting for both the 12:12 and 16:8 plans, further adjustments can be made, provided that the consistency in adhering to the fasting window remains. For example, eating from 3 pm to 11 pm is acceptable and recommended if you work late hours, though it is important to stick with the fasting period of 11 pm to 3 pm the following day.

18:6 Intermittent Fasting Plan

The 18:6 plan is a minor shift from the 16:8 plan, and an easy one to switch to, once you've become comfortable with 16-hour fasts. It requires an additional 2 hours of fasting, which can simply be added to the end or beginning of your current schedule, or with one hour added onto each end of the window. This plan reduces the eating window to six hours, which essentially eliminates one of the three traditional meals. In order to adjust to this shorter time frame for meals, it may be beneficial to have three light meals within the six hours than two larger ones. This will provide more coverage during this window.

The 18-hour fast brings your body closer to reaching a state of ketosis, especially if your meals during the six hours are low carb and low glucose. During a fast, you will naturally become depleted in carbohydrates, which also moves you towards autophagy. While there is a variance in how and when autophagy is reached, as it varies depending on each individual, it can begin around 18 hours for some people and require a longer period of fasting for others. For this reason, this plan can be yet another stepping-stone towards a longer fast in the future.

<u>18:6 Plan A:</u>

This fasting plan begins on a Sunday evening after 1 pm, with the fasting "window" or time period during which there is no food or drink, and ending the following morning at 7 am, when breakfast is served.

Day of the week	Sunday	Monday	Tuesday	Wednesday	Thursday	Friday	Saturday
Feeding or eating window	7 am to 1 pm (includes breakfast with options mid-morning snack and lunch)	7 am to 1 pm	7 am to 1 pm	7 am to 1 pm	7 am to 1 pm	7 am to 1 pm	7 am to 1 pm
Fasting window	1 pm to 7 am the next	1 pm to 7 am the next	1 pm to 7 am the next	1 pm to 7 am the next morni	1 pm to 7 am the next	1 pm to 7 am the next	1 pm to 7 am the next

	morning	morning	morning	ng	morning	morning	morning

An early start is a good option for this plan, concentrating the meals within the first six hours of the day. If you begin your working day later, eating highly nutritious meals within this time frame will provide a good source of fuel, allowing the body to seek sources of stored fats and other options once the energy is used from the previous meals.

In general, it is best to increase the nutrient density of your foods as your eating window shrinks, as there is a longer time period between meals once the fasting begins. While there are no specific meal plans for standard intermittent fasting, keeping the carbs and sugars low, while the protein, healthy fats and nutrients are high, will give your body and cells all that is needed to function well during a fasting window.

<u>18:6 Plan B:</u>

This fasting plan begins on a Sunday evening after 4 pm, allowing for a later start time the following morning at 10 am. A mid-morning beginning provides for a late breakfast or mid-morning snack to break the fast, followed by a standard lunch between 12-1 pm and a light dinner or healthy snack between 3-4 pm.

Day of the week	Sunday	Monday	Tuesday	Wednesday	Thursday	Friday	Saturday
Feeding or eating window	10 am to 4 pm (mid-morning snack, lunch and early dinner 3-4 pm)	10 am to 4 pm	10 am to 4 pm	10 am to 4 pm	10 am to 4 pm	10 am to 4 pm	10 am to 4 pm
Fasting window	4 pm to 10 am the next morning	4 pm to 10 am the next morning	4 pm to 10 am the next morning	4 pm to 10 am the next morning	4 pm to 10 am the next morning	4 pm to 10 am the next morning	4 pm to 10 am the next morning

Once you adapt to shorter eating windows, the rules of breakfast, lunch, and dinner can be eliminated. For the purpose of following an easy plan, mid-morning, mid-afternoon and/or snack options are referenced in plans with shorter windows for eating. These can be considered by their traditional meal names, especially if they are taken around these times, though with intermittent fasting eating windows of 6 hours or less, usually one meal is skipped altogether in order to "fit" within the time frame.

<u>18:6 Plan C:</u>

This fasting plan begins on a Sunday evening after 7 pm, following a hearty dinner, with a breaking of the fast the following afternoon at or shortly after 1 pm. This is the perfect plan for skipping breakfast within the 6-hour window while maintaining two traditional meals (lunch and dinner). A mid-afternoon snack between 3-4 pm, followed by dinner between 6-7 pm works well within this plan. Lunch can be taken anytime after 1 pm.

Day of the week	Sunday	Monday	Tuesday	Wednesday	Thursday	Friday	Saturday
Feeding or eating	1 pm to 7 pm	1 pm to 7 pm	1 pm to 7 pm	1 pm to 7 pm	1 pm to 7 pm	1 pm to 7 pm	1 pm to 7 pm

windo w	(lunch , mid-aftern oon snack, late dinner)						
Fastin g windo w	7 pm to 1 pm the next morni ng	7 pm to 1 pm the next mor ning	7 pm to 1 pm the next mor ning	7 pm to 1 pm the next morni ng	7 pm to 1 pm the next morn ing	7 pm to 1 pm the next mor ning	7 pm to 1 pm the next mor ning

Many people prefer to stay with the 18:6 plan, as it provides a beneficial weight-loss plan. It may or may not provide a path to autophagy or ketosis, depending on the types of foods consumed during the eating window. To reach autophagy, the best option is to expand the fasting window, when it is comfortable to so. This can be a gradual shift from six to five hours a day, for a 19:5 plan, then moving to 20:4, which is the next milestone.

20:4 Intermittent Fasting Plan

The 20:4 fasting plan is often the option many people choose before "jumping" into a full 24-hour fast. As with all fasting methods, take it gradually until you reach this stage, as a 20-hour fast can be a significant change for many. This plan essentially reduces the eating window to four hours, which provides a few options: focus on one meal and supplement with a smaller, lighter meal, or enjoy two full meals at the very beginning of the eating window, and another towards the last half hour. Regardless of how this plan is approached, it greatly reduces meal options, which makes planning a major factor in success.

On a positive note, a 20-hour fast can bring the onset of autophagy for some people. The two-hour increase from an 18-hour fast to 20 hours can be significant in this stage, as autophagy usually begins anywhere between 18-24 hours, which is also a variable and highly contingent on each individual eating plan. Within this range of time, there is a "peak" period where ketosis and autophagy are at their most effective state.

Another advantage of the four-hour plan is the versatility in when to begin and end the eating window. This plan can be switched weekly or every 2-3 weeks to adjust according to preference and schedule. If you have a special occasion or other event planned, including a vacation, shifting the 4-hour window to a later time frame to capture a special meal is available. For the first sample plan below, the four hours begin early in the day, to focus on getting the most out of nutrients and food early for the remainder of the day, and throughout the fasting window:

<u>20:4 Plan A:</u>

This fasting plan begins late Sunday morning and lasts until the following morning at 7 am. The focus on this plan is on a nutrient-rich, high energy meal and supplement within the morning hours, so that there is a good amount of sustenance for the remainder of the day, during the fasting window. The focus for this plan on breakfast, with a mid-morning option for a supplement or snack. To avoid hunger pangs early into the fasting window, breakfast can be taken later, between 10-11 am, and a light snack between 7-7:30am.

Day of the week	Sunda y	Mon day	Tues day	Wedne sday	Thur sday	Frid ay	Satur day
Feedin g or eating windo w	7 am to 11 am (inclu des breakf	7 am to 11 am	7 am to 11 am	7 am to 11 am	7 am to 11 am	7 am to 11 am	7 am to 11 am

	ast with options mid-morning snack)						
Fasting window	1 pm to 7 am the next morning	1 pm to 7 am the next morning	1 pm to 7 am the next morning	1 pm to 7 am the next morning	1 pm to 7 am the next morning	1 pm to 7 am the next morning	1 pm to 7 am the next morning

This plan can be slightly adjusted to begin earlier, at 5 or 6 am, and ending four hours later, at 9 or 10 am.

20:4 Plan B:

This fasting plan begins mid-afternoon on Sunday, ending the following day in the late morning. An early 4-hour window, as illustrated in 20:4 plan A may be too restrictive for many people, who wish to include a later meal before starting the fast.

Day of the	Sunday	Monday	Tuesday	Wednesday	Thursday	Friday	Saturday

week							
Feeding or eating window	10 am to 2 pm (includes breakfast or mid-morning snack with lunch)	10 am to 2 pm	10 am to 2 pm	10 am to 2 pm	10 am to 2 pm	10 am to 2 pm	10 am to 2 pm
Fasting window	2 pm to 10 am the next morning	2 pm to 10 am the next morning	2 pm to 10 am the next morning	2 pm to 10 am the next morning	2 pm to 10 am the next morning	2 pm to 10 am the next morning	2 pm to 10 am the next morning

The most beneficial aspect of this plan is the inclusion of both breakfast and lunch if desired. This schedule is also an option to one full meal, plus a lighter meal with an additional supplement.

During this shorter eating window, it's strongly recommended to eat protein and fat-rich foods that can provide fuel over the next day. Breaking a fast after a window is completed may tempt some people to overeat. This can be avoided by planning and preparing a meal that will digest slowly, such as lean meats, tofu or tempeh and dark green vegetables high in iron and protein (all of which contain fiber). Unless your diet consists of low carb foods only, there is the option of including whole fruits and/or vegetables high in carbs, but also high in potassium and fiber, which offset the effects that carbohydrates have on the body. This fuel will be used up quickly during the fasting window. Examples of healthy foods that contain moderately high carbohydrates include sweet potatoes, bananas, and cherries.

<u>20:4 Plan C:</u>

The third sample option for fasting four hours each day begins at lunch until close to dinner. There is an option of including lunch and skipping dinner for a mid-afternoon snack or splitting two smaller, equal-sized meals within the eating window.

Day of the wee	Sund ay	Mond ay	Tues day	Wedne sday	Thurs day	Frida y	Satur day

k							
Feeding or eating window	12 pm to 4 pm (includes lunch or early afternoon snack with dinner)	12 pm to 4 pm	12 pm to 4 pm	12 pm to 4 pm	12 pm to 4 pm	12 pm to 4 pm	12 pm to 4 pm
Fasting window	4 pm to 12 pm the next afternoon	4 pm to 12 pm the next afternoon	4 pm to 12 pm the next afternoon	4 pm to 12 pm the next afternoon	4 pm to 12 pm the next afternoon	4 pm to 12 pm the next afternoon	4 pm to 12 pm the next afternoon

The focus of this window, from 12-4 pm, can be placed on lunch as the main meal, with a supplement or light early dinner meal between 3-4 pm. Once the fasting window begins at 4 pm, eating a good amount of healthy, whole foods within the four hours will give you enough to sustain your body with nutrients until the following day at noon. Even where your body becomes low on fuel, which will occur during ketosis, and during autophagy, including all the daily nutrient requirements within the four hours is essential to providing your body with a healthy start before fasting begins.

<u>20:4 Plan D:</u>

The final sample option for fasting four hours each day begins after lunch and focuses on the traditional dinner time for the main meal of the day. This plan can implement a hearty meal between 4-6, followed by a lighter, healthy snack between 7-8 pm. Since this eating window starts very late into the day, it's a recommended plan for people who sleep late and begin their day either later in the morning or towards the afternoon. One example of people who will benefit are shift workers or those who generally work evenings or later hours.

Day of the week	Sunday	Monday	Tuesday	Wednesday	Thursday	Friday	Saturday
Feeding or eating	4 pm to 8 pm	4 pm to 8 pm	4 pm to 8 pm	4 pm to 8 pm	4 pm to 8 pm	4 pm to 8 pm	4 pm to 8 pm

window	(includes lunch or early afternoon snack with dinner)						
Fasting window	8 pm to 4 pm the next day	8 pm to 4 pm the next day	8 pm to 4 pm the next day	8 pm to 4 pm the next day	8 pm to 4 pm the next day	8 pm to 4 pm the next day	8 pm to 4 pm the next day

Considering all four of the sample plans, and any number of variations in between, changes can be easily shifted to adjust from one plan to another where it is most suitable. A rotating schedule of different plans may also work for some people, such as 4-8 pm for week one, followed by 12-4 pm for week two, and so on. Most people will adjust to the four-hour fast within a week, though working towards a 6-hour or 8-hour eating window is the best strategy before starting a four-hour window, and especially before diving into a full day or 24-hour fast.

24-Hour Fasting Plan

The full-day fast is an ideal way to reach your autophagy goal, and it is a powerful way to lose weight and maintain consistent weight management on an ongoing basis. While it may seem like an extreme fasting method, it is not recommended for everyone; consulting a doctor or medical professional should be done before starting this method. To plan for the 24-hour fasting window, take into consideration the following:

- Fasting for a full 24 hours should be done only twice or three times weekly at the most. During regular meal planning in between full-day fasts, make sure you include as many whole, healthy foods as possible.

- If you feel faint or weak at any point during a fast, whether it is a duration of 24 hours or less, make sure to have some water and contact a health professional if you have a medical condition that may be impacted by fasting. If needed, break the fast with a light snack and drink some water.

- Drink plenty of water to ensure you have enough hydration during the fast. There is another method of fasting called "dry" fasting, which is more restrictive and does not include any liquid, including water. While dry fasting can be particularly effective in beginning autophagy, it is best to practice in shorter time frames before extending to one full day, so that your body becomes accustomed to the effects of abstaining from food and water.

- Get plenty of rest. This applies to all forms of fasting. A good night's sleep is essential in using your body's nutrient stores for important building and repairs to your brain, cells, and tissues.

24-Hour Fasting (Two days a week): Plan A

To begin your first 24-hour fasting plan, try just two days each week. This may seem like a different path from the 18:6, 20:4 daily intermittent fasting plans that precede this one, though taking a full day off from food consumption should not be taken lightly. The first sample option, below, designates two days for a full 24-hour fast: day 1 as Sunday and day 2 as Wednesday. The positioning of these days allows for equal distribution between both fasting days, allowing for 2-3 days of regular eating in between.

Day of the	Sunda y	Mon day	Tues day	Wedne sday	Thur sday	Frid ay	Satur day

week							
Fasting and/or eating window (24 hours)	Fasting from 9 am until the next day (Day 1 of fasting)	Breakfast at 9am for breakfast	Regular eating	Fasting from 9 am until the next day (Day 2 of fasting)	Breakfast at 9am for breakfast	Regular eating	Regular eating

Options for this plan include shifting the hours to different start and end times. Plan A allows for breakfast prior to 9am before beginning the fast, with a breaking of the fast the following day after 9am. If you begin work earlier than 9am during the week, the start and end time for the fasting window can be moved earlier to 7 or 8am. The same can be done for a later start time, as illustrated in the second sample, plan B.

<u>24-Hour Fasting (Two days a week): Plan B</u>

In the second sample, the two fasting days are altered to begin at lunch, allowing for more time in the morning for a full breakfast, with the option of a light mid-morning snack before beginning a fast at 12 noon. On the following day, the fast is broken at the same time for lunch. This works well with more schedules, as lunch doesn't fluctuate as much as breakfast, which can be anywhere from 5am to 9am for many people, while lunch tends to center around noon.

Day of the week	Sunday	Monday	Tuesday	Wednesday	Thursday	Friday	Saturday
Fasting and/or eating window (24 hours)	Fasting from 12 pm until the next day (Day 1 of fasting)	Breakfast at 12 pm for lunch	Regular eating	Fasting from 12 pm, following breakfast until the next day (Day 2 of fasting)	Breakfast at 12 pm for lunch	Regular eating	Regular eating

A 24-hour, twice-weekly fasting schedule can be increased to three days a week, as long as a full day of regular eating is scheduled in between each fasting day: for each 24-hour fasting period, there should be a minimum of 24 hours of regular eating following the full day fast.

<u>24-Hour Fasting (Three days a week): Plan C</u>

Three 24-hour days of fasting will give you more opportunities to benefit from autophagy on a more regular basis while getting the most out of ketosis during the fasting days.

Day of the week	Sunday	Monday	Tuesday	Wednesday	Thursday	Friday	Saturday
Fasting and/or eating window (24 hours)	Fasting from 12 pm until the next day (Day 1 of	Breakfast at 12 pm for lunch (regular eating resu	Fasting from 12 pm, following breakfast until the	Breakfast at 12 pm for lunch	Regular eating	Fasting from 12 pm, following breakfast until the	Breakfast at 12 pm for lunch (regular eating resumes for 24

	fasting)	mes for 24 hours until the next day)	next day (Day 2 of fasting)			next day (Day 3 of fasting)	hours until the next day)

This sample plan starts at 12 pm, three times a week. Due to the seven days each week, there may be an extra day in between two of the fasting days, with exactly 24 hours of regular eating in between the others. The first day of fasting, day 1, begins after 12 pm on Sunday, with a break the following day, Monday, after 12. A period of 24 hours begins from 12 pm on Monday until the following day at 12 pm, when the second day of fasting begins and ends on Wednesday at 12 pm. Thursday remains a regular eating day with no fasting. Friday begins the third day or 24 hours of fasting at 12 pm, which breaks the following day at 12 pm, leaving another 24 hours of regular eating until the next fasting period, which begins on the following Sunday at 12 pm.

The two-day or three-day 24-hour fasts can be adjusted to accommodate any schedule, provided a minimum 24 hours of regular eating is scheduled in between each fasting day. While this plan is an excellent way to reach the goal of autophagy, there are two more options that may be considered for either autophagy and/or dietary reasons: alternative day fasting and the 5:2 method.

Alternate Day Fasting

This intermittent fasting method takes the two or three days per week approach and increases the frequency of fasting to every other day, alternating one day of regular eating with one day of fasting, 24 hours for each period. This pattern can be done on a short-term or longer-term basis, provided you have enough nutrients and eat healthy, whole foods with little or no processing or artificial additives. The necessity of implementing healthier, more sustainable foods becomes increasingly more important as fasting windows and frequency expands.

The schedule below provides a guide on how alternate day fasting looks like and how it can be implemented into your regular schedule. The first plan works with the 12 pm to 12 pm option, as offered in the weekly 24-hour fasting samples, and is a good time frame to begin with, as it ensures that you will have at least one meal each day, either before or after 12 pm, depending on which day(s) you start and end each fasting window. Due to the nature of alternate fasting, where every other day of the week will vary from the first to the second week, this plan is shown in a span of two weeks:

Alternate Day Fasting: Plan A

Day of the week (Week 1)	Sunday	Monday	Tuesday	Wednesday	Thursday	Friday	Saturday
Fasting and/or eating window (24 hours)	Fasting from 12 pm until the next day (Day 1 of fasting)	Breakfast at 12 pm for lunch (regular eating resumes for 24 hours until the next	Fasting from 12 pm, following breakfast until the next day (Day 2 of fasting)	Breakfast at 12 pm for lunch (regular eating resumes for 24 hours until the next day)	Fasting from 12 pm, following breakfast until the next day (Day 3 of fasting)	Breakfast at 12 pm for lunch (regular eating resumes for 24 hours until the next day)	Fasting from 12 pm, following breakfast until the next day (Day 4 of fasting)

		day)					
Day of the week (Week 2)	Sunday	Monday	Tuesday	Wednesday	Thursday	Friday	Saturday
Fasting and/ or eating window (24 hours)	Breakfast at 12 pm for lunch (regular eating resumes for 24 hours until the	Fasting from 12 pm, following breakfast until the next day (Day 5 of fasting)	Breakfast at 12 pm for lunch (regular eating resumes for 24 hours until the	Fasting from 12 pm, following breakfast until the next day (Day 6 of fasting)	Breakfast at 12 pm for lunch (regular eating resumes for 24 hours until the	Fasting from 12 pm, following breakfast until the next day (Day 7 of fasting) (Day 3 of	Breakfast at 12 pm for lunch (regular eating resumes for 24 hours until the next day)

	next day)		next day)		next day)	fastin g)	

The fasting days over a 14-day or two-week period are scheduled as follows:

- Sunday (day 1, week 1)

- Tuesday (day 3, week 1)

- Thursday (day 5, week 1)

- Saturday (day 7, week 1)

- Monday (day 9, week 2)

- Wednesday (day 11, week 2)

- Friday (day 13, week 2)

On day 14th, or Saturday, the final day of the two weeks, regular eating is resumed at 12 pm, with fasting beginning on the following day at 12 pm as per the first week's schedule. Rotating the two weeks to accommodate alternate days of fasting with eating can be adjusted to begin on either the first or second day of week one and follow accordingly. The next plan provides an earlier start time to allow for an earlier breakfast.

<u>Alternate Day Fasting: Plan B</u>

Day of the week (Week 1)	Sunday	Monday	Tuesday	Wednesday	Thursday	Friday	Saturday
Fasting and/or eating window (24 hours)	Fasting from 8am until the next day (Day 1 of fasting)	Breakfast at 8am for breakfast (regular eating resumes for 24 hours until the next	Fasting from 8am, following breakfast until the next day (Day 2 of fasting)	Breakfast at 8am for breakfast (regular eating resumes for 24 hours until the next day)	Fasting from 8am, following breakfast until the next day (Day 3 of fasting)	Breakfast at 8am for breakfast (regular eating resumes for 24 hours until the next day)	Fasting from 8am, following breakfast until the next day (Day 4 of fasting)

		day)					
Day of the week (Week 2)	Sunday	Monday	Tuesday	Wednesday	Thursday	Friday	Saturday
Fasting and/ or eating window (24 hours)	Breakfast at 8am for breakfast (regular eating resumes for 24 hours until	Fasting from 8am, following breakfast until the next day (Day 5 of fasting)	Breakfast at 8am for breakfast (regular eating resumes for 24 hours until	Fasting from 8am, following breakfast until the next day (Day 6 of fasting)	Breakfast at 8am for breakfast (regular eating resumes for 24 hours until	Fasting from 8am, following breakfast until the next day (Day 7 of fasting)	Breakfast at 8am for breakfast (regular eating resumes for 24 hours until the next

	the next day)		the next day)		the next day)		day)

The second sample plan follows the exact same idea as plan A, with a shift from 12 pm to 8am. This is an ideal method of fasting for schedules that require an earlier meal taken either before the fasting begins (before 8am) and once the window ends (just after 8am the following morning). The third and final option displays how a later start would look like over a two-week period, beginning at 4 pm.

<u>Alternate Day Fasting: Plan C</u>

Day of the week (Week 1)	Sunday	Monday	Tuesday	Wednesday	Thursday	Friday	Saturday
Fasting and/ or eating wind	Fasting from 4 pm until the next	Breakfast at 4 pm for dinner	Fasting from 4 pm, following a late	Breakfast at 4 pm for dinner (regular	Fasting from 4 pm, following a late	Breakfast at 4 pm for dinner (regul	Fasting from 4 pm, following a late

ow (24 hours)	day (Day 1 of fasting)	(regular eating resumes for 24 hours until the next day)	lunch or mid-afternoon snack until the next day (Day 2 of fasting)	eating resumes for 24 hours until the next day)	lunch or mid-afternoon snack until the next day (Day 3 of fasting)	ar eating resumes for 24 hours until the next day)	lunch or mid-afternoon snack until the next day (Day 4 of fasting)
Day of the week (Week 2)	Sunday	Monday	Tuesday	Wednesday	Thursday	Friday	Saturday
Fasting and/ or eating g	Breakfast at 4 pm for dinn	Fasting from 4 pm, following	Breakfast at 4 pm for dinne	Fasting from 4 pm, following a late	Breakfast at 4 pm for dinne	Fasting from 4 pm, following a	Breakfast at 4 pm for dinne

wind ow (24 hours)	er (regu lar eatin g resu mes for 24 hour s until the next day)	a late lunch or mid- after noon snack until the next day (Day 5 of fastin g)	r (regu lar eatin g resu mes for 24 hour s until the next day)	lunch or mid- aftern oon snack until the next day (Day 6 of fasting)	r (regu lar eatin g resu mes for 24 hour s until the next day)	late lunch or mid- aftern oon snack until the next day (Day 7 of fastin g)	r (regu lar eatin g resu mes for 24 hours until the next day)

All alternate day fasting samples are beneficial in the same way, with the only difference being preference and schedule. If alternating days becomes too much, changing back to twice a week for 24 hours or a 20:4 or 18:6 plan may be a better option. While intermittent fasting is beneficial for many people, it can present challenges for some and is not the best method for everyone.

Extended Fasting for Periods of Over 24 Hours

Once you have mastered 24-hour fasting and wish to extend your level of fast to yet another milestone, there are extended options of over 24 hours. Typically, this is done less frequently, to allow your body to recover from abstaining from food for over one day, or up to 3 days in total. Extended periods of fasting, if followed correctly, will provide the benefits of autophagy and ketosis within the first 24 hours. Any extension of the fasting period will continue the benefits of both, though the peak or desired point of maximum effectiveness for both ketosis and autophagy will decline after 24 hours. For this reason, fasting longer than 24 hours is not necessarily required, though it can provide additional health benefits, such as detoxification and significant weight loss within a short period of time. Once you are prepared to embark on a long fast of 30, 48 or 60 hours or more, plan to ensure you have a stress-free environment and support available before you begin:

- Speak to your family, friends, doctor, and/or anyone else who will be directly affected by your extended fast and may be able to provide support, encouragement, and/or advice.

- Rule out any medical conditions that may worsen or negatively impact your health during a long-term fast.

- Avoid beginning a fast during a stressful time or when there is a special occasion. It is during exceptional circumstances and event that we may want to break the fast and/or enjoy a meal that will occur during the fasting window.

- If you work a standard five days each week, Monday through Friday, plan an extended fast over a weekend to minimize temptation at work to eat

- Spend as much time as possible in a calming, natural environment to get the most out of the experience. Fasting shouldn't be considered a chore or unpleasant, but rather, a rest from eating and other activities that increase stress. If there is the option of spending a weekend away in the countryside or somewhere else natural and relaxing, this will greatly improve your chances of success.

- Keep a diary of your experience and take note of any sensations, side effects, or experiences of your fasting journey. This will help you to identify any concerns and/or challenges that can be addressed

- Exercise mindfully. High impact exercise is excellent for a regular dieting and short term fasting, though should be used with caution during extended periods of fasting. For this reason, begin slowly and gently, adding yoga, Pilates and/or other gently guided methods of stretching and moving that will keep your body fit while giving you more relaxation

- Get a massage. Every now and again, whether we have a health condition requiring massage therapy or not, it can be an excellent way to work through and minimize our body's stress, especially during periods of fasting.

How long should I fast? It depends on your goal. Athletes and people who tend to be very active will take a long fast, between 60-72 hours (up to three days) to maximize burning fat stores and losing weight fast, while continuing to exercise and build lean muscle mass. It is during this process where autophagy begins to break down old cellular matter, once all other sources of energy have been exhausted, in order to repair and rebuild in the body. This process makes our bodies more efficient, and just one reason why more athletes are implementing a fasting plan into their diet to gain the benefits of autophagy.

The chart below indicates how scheduling a 30-hour fast can take place over a period of two days, from Sunday at 12 pm until the following day, Monday, at 6pm. Since the 30-hour period is slightly longer than 24 hours, it may be possible to fast for this duration of time once per week, though once every 2-4 weeks is beneficial and allows for plenty of time to recover from the extended time frame.

30-Hour Fasting Plan

Day of the week	Sunday	Monday	Tuesday	Wednesday	Thursday	Friday	Saturday
Fasting period (over one day) and regular eating	Fasting begins at 12 pm	Fasting until 6pm (completing a 30 hour fast)	Regular eating	Regular eating	Regular eating	Regular eating	Regular eating

The next sample plan shows how a 48-hour or two full days of fasting may be scheduled during a regular week.

48-Hour Fasting Plan

Day of the week	Sunday	Monday	Tuesday	Wednesday	Thursday	Friday	Saturday
Fasting period (over one day) and regular eating	Fasting begins at 12 pm	Fasting continues	Fasting continues until 12 pm, completing a full 48 hours	Regular eating	Regular eating	Regular eating	Regular eating

The two-day fast begins similarly to the 30-hour fast, at noon or 12 pm on one day, continuing for the next day (Monday), then ending on Tuesday at 12 pm. A 48-hour fast should be done no more than once every two weeks, and preferably just once monthly. If you wish to benefit more often from fasting, it's best to implement smaller, more frequent intermittent fasting options before and after a long-term fast, allowing for one full day on either end (before and after) of the extended fast.

Increasing the fasting window longer, to 60 or 72 hours should not be done more than once a month. Extended fasting for any length of time after 24 hours should be done carefully to ensure that enough healthy foods are consumed just prior to and immediately following the fast. Breaking a fast, especially after a long-term session, should be done first with a light, easy to digest meal, to avoid any possible indigestion or other issues.

The following two plans, for 60 hours and 72 hours, indicate how these long-term fasts can be scheduled in a one-week time, though should only be done once every month or every two months:

<u>60-Hour Fasting Plan</u>

Day of the week	Sunday	Monday	Tuesday	Wednesday	Thursday	Friday	Saturday
Fasting period (over one day) and regul	Fasting begins at 12 pm	Fasting continues	Fasting continues until 6pm, completing a full	Regular eating	Regular eating	Regular eating	Regular eating

ar eatin g			60 hours				

This 60-hour schedule provides a partial day of fasting beginning on Sunday, followed by a full day on Monday, with a break in fasting at dinner time on Tuesday. The fasting period is essentially two and a half days long.

<u>72-Hour Fasting Plan</u>

The 72-hour fast, which is three full days, is the longest recommended fast. Any fasting for longer than three days can cause weakness and other symptoms, if not properly prepared for. While an extended fast can be rewarding, it also requires staying in tune with your body's needs and paying attention to any symptoms that may cause more harm than good. During your fast, take time for yourself to meditate, stretch, and rest in order to get the most out of this state. It's a time to reflect on your goals and reasons for fasting and taking comfort in the positive outcome.

Dry Fasting Versus Wet (or Regular) Fasting

During a fast, water and a limited amount of liquids that do not increase or affect your glucose levels, may be consumed as needed. The benefits of fasting will not be adversely affected by drinking water and other permissible liquids, and ketosis will be achieved in the exact same way with or without liquids. The reason for dry fasting is due to how much quickly cell regeneration can be achieved through autophagy, a state that is reached sooner when all foods and liquids are abstained from altogether. This form of fasting should be done with careful consideration to avoid dehydration. Dry fasting is practiced for religious and spiritual reasons, for short, intermittent periods or longer, expanded time frames. If you plan on dry fasting, any and all of the above intermittent fasting plans, including more extended periods apply. Start with a short time frame, and gradually increase over time, until you reach the desired plan to achieve your objective. Keep the following tips in mind when dry fasting:

- Avoid high impact exercise that will dehydrate the body quickly. While exercise of any kind is beneficial during a regular or "wet" fast, it should be limited if liquids are not consumed. Low impact movement, such as stretching and walking, are the best options during a dry fast

- Monitor how you feel, especially your energy levels. If you have the option of taking a day off work or minimizing your tasks for the day, it can provide a good opportunity to focus on the moment. At any time if you begin to feel weak or sick, sipping a bit of water may be an option to avoid getting ill. Usually, this is not an issue, and most people get through a dry fast with little to no problems. There will be some symptoms associated with feeling tired, hungry, and thirsty, though they are temporary and will come and go during the fasting window.

- Dry fasting is not for everyone. If you don't succeed the first time, try again, or simply stick with other forms of fasting that allow for liquids and small periods of time.

5:2 Fasting Method

The 5:2 method is different than all other forms of fasting, in that it allows for some food consumption during the fasting window. This method consists of five days of regular eating and two days of fasting or consuming food and drink of up to 500 calories only. During the regular days, there are no carb or calorie restrictions, though eating low carb is an option. The two days of fasting are spread across the week, to ensure at least one full day of regular eating falls within both days.

The 5:2 fasting plan can vary from week to week, depending on personal preference and schedule. The advantage of this plan is the flexibility, and the allowance of some food and drink consumption during the fasting days. The following schedule is a sample of how this plan can be organized in a typical week:

5:2 Fasting Schedule: Plan A

Day of the week	Sun day	Monda y	Tues day	Wedn esday	Thur sday	Friday	Satur day
5:2 meth od (two days	Reg ular eati ng	Fastin g (eating up to 500	Reg ular eati ng	Fastin g (eating up to 500	Regu lar eatin g	Regul ar eating	Regul ar eatin g

fasting, 5 days regular eating)		calories for the day)		calories for the day)			

The above plan provides just one full day of regular eating in between the two fasting days of the week. The period in between these 500-calorie days can be expanded to two or three days, as shown in plan B and C:

5:2 Fasting Schedule: Plan B

Day of the week	Sunday	Monday	Tuesday	Wednesday	Thursday	Friday	Saturday
5:2 method (two days fasting, 5	Regular eating	Fasting (eating up to 500 calories for	Regular eating	Regular eating	Fasting (eating up to 500 calori	Regular eating	Regular eating

days regul ar eatin g)		the day)			es for the day)		

The second plan (above) allows for two days of regular eating in between fasting, while the third option provides three days in between during the week, with one fasting day on Sunday, and the other on a Thursday.

5:2 Fasting Schedule: Plan C

Day of the week	Sunda y	Mon day	Tues day	Wedn esday	Thurs day	Frida y	Satur day
5:2 meth od (two days fasti ng, 5 days regul	Fastin g (eatin g up to 500 calori es for the day)	Regu lar eatin g	Reg ular eati ng	Regula r eating	Fastin g (eatin g up to 500 calori es for the	Regul ar eatin g	Regul ar eatin g

ar				day)		
eatin						
g)						

Options for eating during the 500-calorie fasting days include simple foods that provide enough nutrients to supplement the carbs and fat stores your body already contains in order to use during the fasting window:

- One or two boiled eggs (for the duration of the day)

- Small or moderate green salad with a balsamic dressing. Cucumbers, shredded carrots, slivered almonds are among the options to include with spinach, arugula and/or lettuce.

- Bone broth and/or miso soup

- A small portion of fish (tuna or salmon) with salad

- Tea, coffee and lots of water

- Avoid all sugar and sweeteners as much as possible

While the 5:2 fasting method is very beneficial for weight loss and maintenance and reducing or preventing many health conditions and diseases, it's not the most effective method of achieving ketosis or autophagy. This is due to having no window where there is complete avoidance of all food, as in other intermittent or long-term fasting methods. While the body is consuming food, even in small amounts, reaching autophagy is not likely. The 5:2 fasting plan is a good option in between periods of intermittent fasting, where you decide to take a break from traditional fasting completely while keeping your food intake monitored for calories for weight maintenance.

Alternating Between Carb Cycling and Low Carb Eating

Bodybuilders and athletes may often choose to "carb-up" or increase the number of carbohydrates in their diet for certain periods of time, to prepare for marathons, races, and other very physically demanding activities. This may infrequently occur, only a few days or hours prior to such an event, or on an intermittent basis, to match a high impact exercise schedule on certain days, while reducing the carb intake for the remaining days to match lower impact exercise or rest periods. This type of carb "cycling" usually revolves around a ketogenic diet, with the low carb days strictly adhering to the 20 grams or below target, and the higher carb days are increasing to add more fuel for the activities. This type of diet is best suited for experienced athletes who are not looking to lose weight, but rather build muscle and maximize the amount of energy, whether it be carbs or fat, to use for that purpose.

Low to high carb cycling will not achieve autophagy, though once the carbs are fully depleted after a strenuous exercise event, moving into a mode of fasting instead of low carb eating can bring a period of ketosis and result in autophagy soon after. This is due to the body's need for materials to build more muscle and tissue. When food is restricted or abstained from for a period of 18 hours or more following a high carb day and depletion of those carbs as energy, autophagy can be easier to achieve at the 18-hour point. So, while this form of diet isn't the best way to reach autophagy, it can definitely lead to this if intermittent fasting is combined during the low carb part of the cycle.

Other Diets and Methods for Achieving Ketosis and Autophagy

Are there any specific diets and other ways of eating that achieve autophagy? While many paths lead to autophagy, there is no specific one-fits-all diet that will make it work for everyone in the same way. Like diets, not all methods of eating or meal plans work for the individual. For this reason, the ketogenic diet and low carb eating provide a method or way of eating, by reducing the number of carbohydrates, while increasing fats and protein, though without setting strict guidelines on the calories consumed or amount of foods. The ketogenic diet provides a head-start to intermittent fasting, which leads to autophagy, by reducing the carbohydrates in the body prior to fasting. This allows the body to use up its fat stores sooner during a fast and moving onto cell regeneration much sooner. A few points to keep in mind when planning for intermittent fasting that leads to autophagy:

- Become familiar with foods that are low in carbs and make them a regular part of your diet, even if you do not plan on committing to a ketogenic diet on a full-time basis; you can begin to restrict carbs on a gradual basis to prepare ahead.

- Drink water when you feel hungry. Most hunger pangs are symptoms of thirst, and drinking plenty of water will help reduce overeating as well as eating the wrong foods

- Stay active. Exercise and engage in regular movement to maintain and regulate your metabolism. It also keeps your body in an accelerated state of burning carbs, followed by fat stores, which is a quicker way to becoming fat-adapted, where your body switches into ketosis and burns fat as its main fuel. This is a good way to prepare for intermittent fasting and further towards autophagy.

Every person's body varies in response to intermittent fasting and the different types of diets that support ketosis and reducing carbs. Try different methods to determine which works best for your body and goals and avoid any methods that don't yield the results you want to achieve.

Chapter 5: The Horizon of Autophagy

Autophagy is a fascinating tool that we can switch on in our bodies to replenish and rejuvenate our cells, which are the basic building blocks of our body. Cells are continually dying and regenerating within our bodies, and as we age, the regeneration of cells slows down, where fewer cells are replacing the ones that die off. As a result, our body processes slow down as there are fewer cells to do the same work required to function. While increasing the number of cells is simply not possible or available, improving the quality of the fewer new cells that replace, the older ones, is paramount to maintaining excellent health and slowing down the aging process. Effectively, quality will take the place of quantity. With fewer cells, your body can continue to function exceptionally well, as long as only good quality cells and tissues develop on an ongoing basis.

At which point does autophagy occur? The first step is to determine at which point ketosis begins, which is the switch from burning carbs or glucose as fuel to stores of fat. When this occurs, your body is using up the fat as fuel because there are no carbs left to use. During this time, cellular repair and rebuilding are continually in process, and the body will find any sources possible to accomplish this goal. The chart below indicates the approximate decrease in plasma insulin in the body during various points of a fast, in increments of 6 hours, starting at twelve hours of fasting. According to the chart, insulin steadily decreases between 12 and 24 hours, from just above 60 to around 40 pmol/L of insulin. After 24 hours, the insulin levels begin to increase, in part due to the body's production of glucose. This occurs during ketosis when the body produces ketones in response to low glucose levels. From 24 hours to 48, there is an increase, followed by a decrease at 48 hours or a second "peak." After this point, the levels rise towards 60 hours.

There are basically two peak periods within the 60-hour fasting period illustrated in the chart: the first at 24 hours and a second peak around 48 hours. As this is an approximate gauge used for reference, it should be noted that the levels can vary considerably if you employ low carb eating prior to fasting and/or dry fasting, at least during the first 18-24 hours of an extended fast. The second chart below is a simplified version of the same chart, with similar results, indicating a peak or ideal goal of 24 hours for shifting into autophagy, where the body must search for the old, damaged cellular matter to break down and reuse for building and repairing materials in the production of new cells.

The general direction of achieving autophagy indicates a 24-hour fast as the ideal period for reaching this goal. The peak "dip" indicated in the basic graph above is the peak point that prevails in most charts and diagrams indicating the onset of autophagy.

What happens when we reach the point of autophagy? This is an important step during which our cells shift towards cleaning up the cellular waste and damaged, broken down matter to rebuild. Our bodies have the ability to detect which materials are damaged and will use these first, avoiding already healthy cells and tissues available. When this process begins, at the 24-hour mark, we have several options:

- Continue fasting to continue the benefit the cellular rejuvenation process. As the graphs indicate, this process will continue, on a somewhat consistent level for a period of time, following the first 24 hours

- Break your fast. Autophagy may begin before 24 hours, if your method is dry fasting, and/or if your eating plan includes a significant reduction in carbs and glucose, for at least 24 hours prior to fasting

- Enjoy some bone broth and/or gradually break your fast. This will stop the production of autophagosomes, though it will also infuse a significant amount of nutrients to support your body

Determining when autophagy begins remains vague, with little to no indication of when it begins. Unless we can test our bodies for the presence of autophagosome production, we can only rely on the general guidelines that will lead our bodies to this point, and measure ketones to confirm ketosis as a means to determine that we are close to achieving this goal. Overall, using intermittent fasting along with a low carb or ketogenic diet, is the best way to reach the goal of autophagy and all of its benefits.

Chapter 6: Foods and Nutrients That Support Autophagy and Ketosis

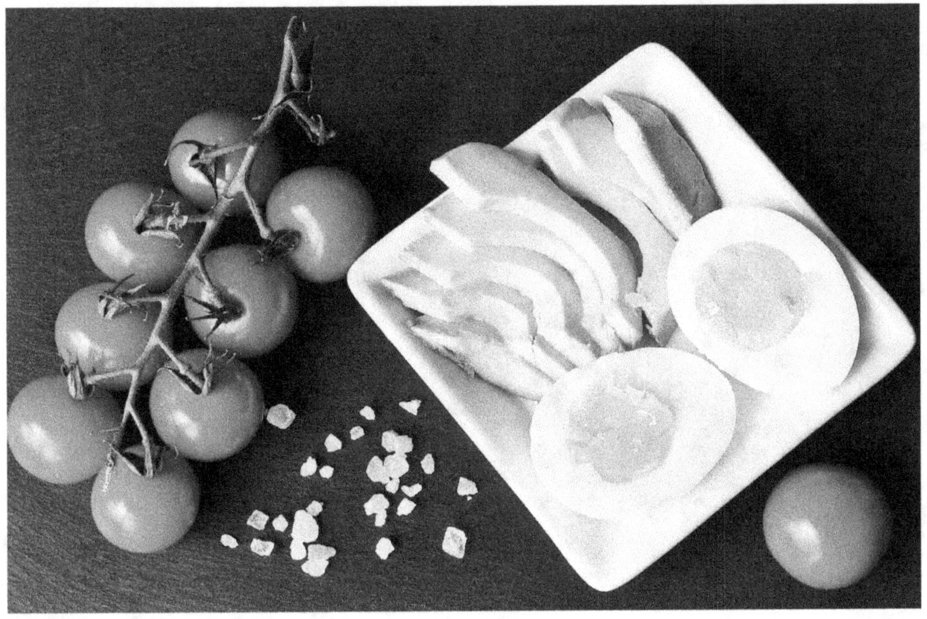

The ketogenic diet is the best way to achieve ketosis while supporting the effectiveness of intermittent fasting to gain amazing benefits of autophagy. Planning meals and funding recipes with low carbs and low glycemic levels doesn't have to be difficult. Most food options are usually available locally and within a reasonable budget. This section focuses on the best options for simple foods that can be used as a foundation to build your diet.

Simple, Key Foods for Ketogenic or Low Carb Diet

Eggs

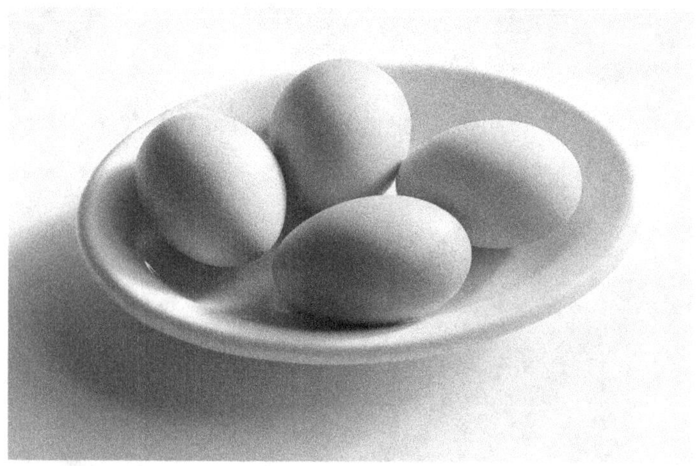

A popular breakfast option, eggs are a good option any time of day within your eating window. They can be prepared in different ways for convenience (boiled or scrambled, for example) and added to almost any meal. On their own, eggs contain enough nutrients to meet some of the daily requirements: omega 3 and 6 fatty acids, protein and calcium are all included in just one serving. Just one or two eggs each day can add a good amount of minerals and fats that your body needs. Eggs are also low in carbohydrates, and glucose, which make them an ideal choice for the ketogenic diet. In baking, eggs are often used and may continue to be included as an ingredient in many recipes, where other items are replaced or modified to accommodate a low carb diet.

Spinach, Kale and Dark Leafy Greens

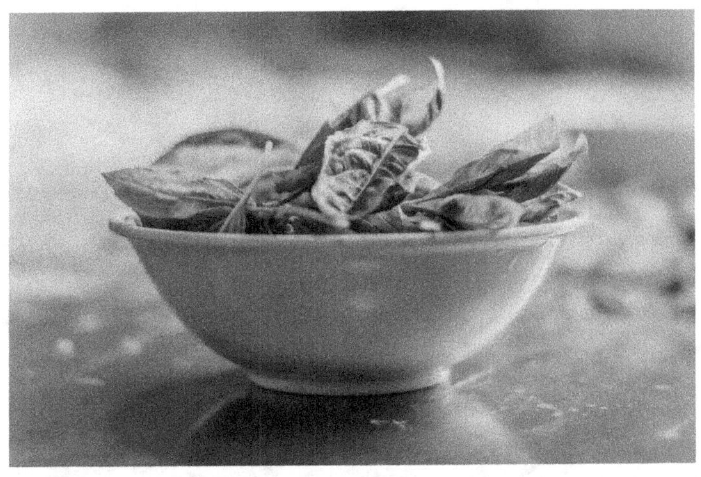

Dark, leafy greens are generally an excellent option because of the rich amount and variety of nutrients they all contain. While there are more dark green leafy options, such as arugula, Swiss chard, and parsley, spinach and kale are often available in most grocery stores and local farmer's markets, which make them easy to include in your diet. Dark greens contain a wealth of vitamins, iron, calcium, and protein. In fact, many vegans and vegetarians can obtain most of their dietary needs from these vegetables. They are most powerful raw when the enzymes remain active, and the nutrients absorbed more thoroughly into the body and used efficiently. These vegetables are also excellent in soups, stir-fries or stews, and can be easily blended into juices and smoothies.

Bone Broth

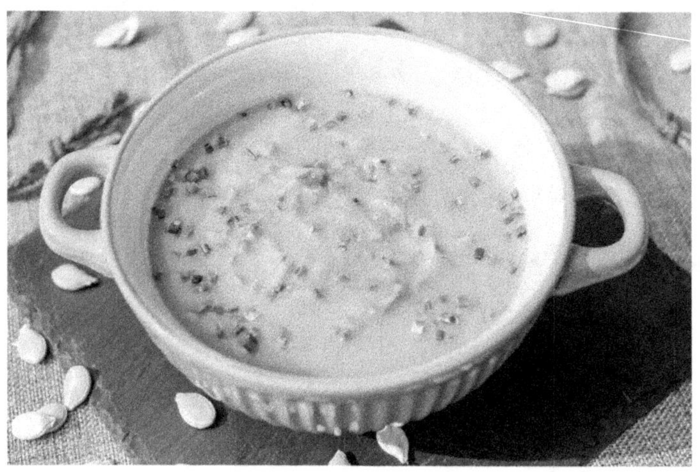

A simple yet very effective way to get most of your nutrients is from bone broth. Chicken and beef are the most common and popular options for these broths. Bone broth can be made from scratch from leftover poultry and beef bones, though the process is time-consuming and can take approximately 24 hours to transfer all of the bones' nutrients into the broth, for maximum nutrition value. For this reason, bone broth can be found in dried powder form for easy preparation, as well as cartons that are ready to heat and serve. Some companies add flavors, such as spices and herbs, to enhance the taste, as broth tends to be very mild and low in flavor. When choosing a broth that is already prepared, be sure to find a good, reputable brand that does not contain preservatives and preferably uses all-natural and organic ingredients.

One of the most important and beneficial ingredients in bone broth is collagen. It is very advantageous to our bone health and provides anti-aging properties as well. Collagen is contained in protein and the main part or component in connective tissue. There are many benefits to taking collagen, whether in bone broth, where is it naturally or in supplement form:

- It reduces joint pain associated with the breakdown of cartilage, as a result of arthritis and similar conditions.

- It is anti-aging in that it promotes better elasticity in skin and tissues

- Reduction in cellulite and toxins stored in the body

- Supports cognitive function and brain health

- Improves digestion and microbial balance (bacterial systems) within the body

If you choose to take collagen as a supplement instead of bone broth, be sure to research the different options available to obtain the most natural, and the best quality available. Bone broth is a convenient and easy way to obtain a lot of nutrients without preparing a complete meal. It's ideal on the go and in between meals. Bone broth can be used during intermittent fasting and as a meal replacement during an eating window if desired.

Berries

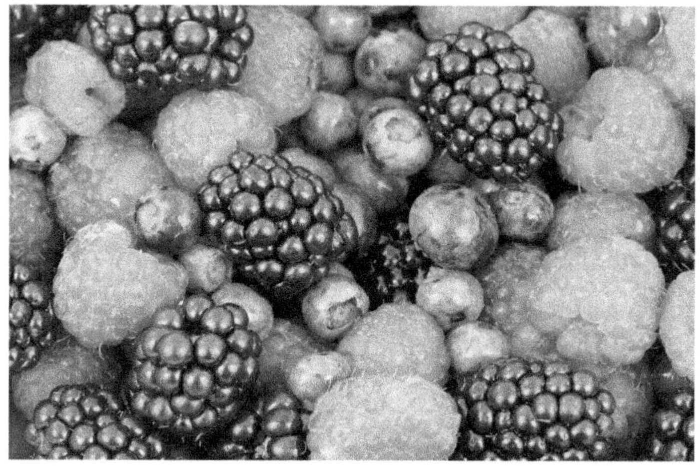

All berries are exceptionally healthy and full of antioxidants, which support the immune system, prevent cancer and other diseases. Strawberries, raspberries, blueberries and blackberries, currants and gooseberries are included in this category, and can be a great snack on their own, served with yogurt or with full fat, sugar-free cream (dairy or non-dairy).

Berries are ideal for smoothies and easy to find when in season at local markets and grocery stores. While fresh berries are the best option, some varieties tend to ripen quickly and need to be consumed within a short period of time. For this reason, frozen berries are a good option for smoothies, desserts and can be kept for longer periods of time for convenient use.

Soy

Tofu, tempeh, miso, and soy products, in general, contain most of our daily nutrients and are an ideal replacement for meat and dairy products. While soy is a great way to increase plant-based protein in your diet, it isn't for everyone, particularly people who have allergies or dietary sensitivities related to soy foods. To minimize risks or side effects of soy, which include bloating and occasional issues with digestion, choose organic, high-quality soy products, preferably from a familiar source or company. Fermented soy foods, such as miso and tempeh, contain the protein, calcium, fiber, and vitamins contained in regular soy products, plus B12, which is rarely found in plant-based foods, and usually only in red meats. Vitamin D is usually found in soy products that are fortified to ensure this essential vitamin is included in your diet.

Seafood and Fatty Fish

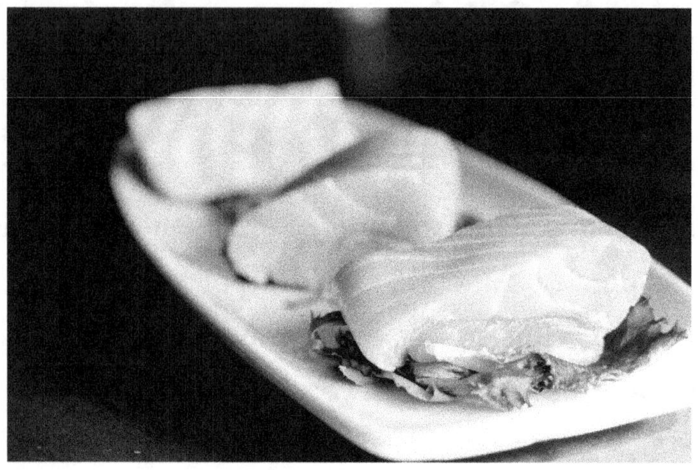

Fish is a good source of healthy fats, protein, and calcium. In a pinch, canned tuna or salmon is a great option to add to a salad or as a side dish. As the main meal, baked or fried fish is a quick way to prepare a dinner or weekend lunch. Even a small portion of fish can be a strong boost to enhance improvements in cognitive function and building muscle. If seafood is not an agreeable option, other meats such as poultry and good quality red meats are good options for increasing iron and protein in your diet.

Sea Vegetables

Kelp and seaweed are examples of sea vegetables that provide a lot of nutrients, such as iron, protein, and various minerals. While they are not always readily available, seaweed has become popular as a snack, in dried sheets, and as a part of sushi cuisine. On its own, seaweed is a good snack option and can be combined with seafood, avocado and/or vegetables for a complete meal.

Avocado

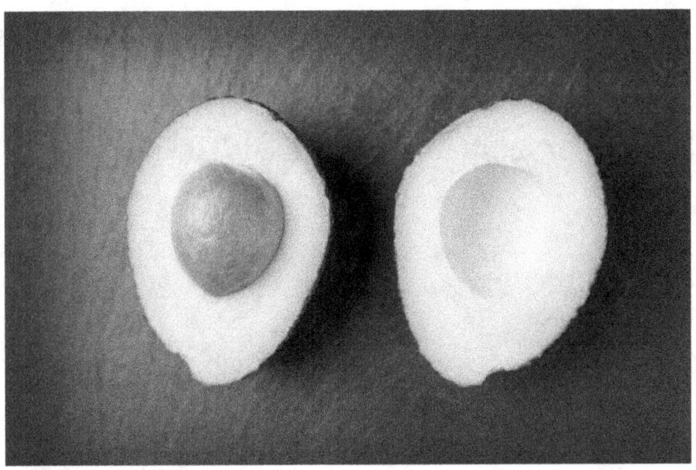

This fruit, which is often mistaken for a vegetable, deserves a category of its own for its numerous benefits. High in fiber, vitamins, and healthy fats, avocado is an ideal food for a low carb or ketogenic diet. It is often considered a superfood because of its high nutrient value. Avocados are filling, and just one serving can complete a meal or snack. They are also excellent as part of a salad, when they are less ripe, or mixed into smoothie, dip or side dish.

Simple Recipes and Meal Suggestions

Scrambled Eggs Skillet

This is a simple, yet effective meal that uses eggs as a base, and adds vegetables, herbs, and other ingredients, as desired, to enhance flavor and add nutrients. An ideal breakfast meal, this dish can be served and enjoyed at any time during your eating window and provides a lot of protein and energy that will last for hours. The ingredients are simple and can be switched and/or replaced, added or omitted as preferred. The recipe below serves 2-3 portions:

- 3-4 eggs (medium or large)

- ½ cup frozen or fresh spinach, sliced in small pieces

- 1 onion, diced into small pieces

- Dried basil, dill, turmeric and/or other spices and/or herbs as desired

- ½ green pepper sliced into small squares, about ½ or smaller

- 2-3 small mushrooms, sliced thinly

- Sea salt and black pepper (to taste)

Heat a skillet on medium and add 1-2 tablespoons of olive oil. In a small bowl, prepare the eggs by whisking them together, then add to the skillet. Stir and scramble the eggs and reduce the heat. Vegetables included in this recipe can be prepared the night before or just prior to scrambling the eggs so that they are ready to add once the eggs are cooked, or while they are cooking. Add the above ingredients in the following order, to get the most out of their flavor and textures:

- Add spices, salt, and pepper with the eggs in the bowl or while they are scrambled in the skillet

- Herbs can also be added during the scrambling process, or with the vegetables

- Add spinach and green peppers, along with other crunchy or hard-textured vegetables, as they take longer to cook

- Add mushrooms and softer ingredients at the end, as minimal cooking is needed

This dish takes about 10 minutes to cook fully, once all ingredients are in the skillet. The following options may also be considered:

- Diced cubes of ham, smoked salmon, pieces of bacon (fried or baked prior to the skillet)

- Asparagus is a delicious option, though it takes longer to cook. For best results, steam asparagus in a small or medium pot until gently softened, then add to the skillet.

- Kale can be substituted for spinach, though it has a rougher texture and can take longer to cook. Extra time should be taken into consideration, or fry or steam kale in advance for an easier mix.

Tofu Scramble Skillet

If you are vegan or looking for an alternative to scrambled eggs, the scrambled egg skillet dish above can be made with tofu as the substitute. This option requires a bit more preparation, to add flavor to the tofu by marinating overnight or several hours before this meal is cooked. The best type of tofu to use is extra firm, with little or no additives, or flavors added. This variety of tofu is fairly common and can be found in most grocery stores. The following ingredients are used in the margination process, which is easy to prepare:

- 1 block of extra firm tofu

- 2 cups of vegetable broth (or enough to cover the block of tofu)

- Herbs, spices, and/or flavors to add. This may include the same spices and herbs used in the egg skillet dish.

- Turmeric is recommended for its nutritional value and pleasant taste. It also adds color to tofu, making it appear more like scrambled eggs.

- Dried bay leaves

Combine all of the ingredients into a medium-sized container that can be sealed and refrigerated. This includes the broth, spices, turmeric, and bay leaves, plus other ingredients as preferred. Pour over the firm tofu or simply add the block to the mixed broth, ensuring there is enough to cover the tofu so that it is fully submerged for marinating. To make it easier, and reduce the amount of broth needed, slice the tofu lengthwise or in large cubes before marinating. The best results of this process require soaking the tofu overnight, though two hours minimum should be sufficient to transfer the bulk of the flavor.

Once the tofu is ready, remove from the fridge and heat the skillet on medium, as you would to scramble eggs. Add olive oil. Drain the broth liquid from the container and retain ¼ or ½ cups to add to the skillet. Mash the tofu in a medium bowl, so that it even, with all pieces of tofu similar in size. Add to the skillet, along with the broth liquid, vegetables and add more spices and herbs as desired.

Options for this dish include adding 1 teaspoon of miso paste to strengthen the flavor. Garlic can also be added.

Shakshuka

Eggs are a feature of this dish, which adds a tomato sauce base, plus herbs and other ingredients. Like the skillet dish, shakshuka can be modified to include or omit ingredients are desired, while retaining the two main ingredients: eggs and tomato sauce. The tomato sauce in this recipe can either be homemade from stewed tomatoes or canned. Canned tomatoes are often the best option for time management, though its best to avoid varieties or brands with added sugars and other preservatives. For this recipe, diced or pureed tomatoes are the best option, as they create a smooth base for poaching eggs. This meal involves just one skillet and can be served directly from the skillet once it is ready or transferred to a deep dish.

To prepare this meal, heat the skillet on medium and add 1-2 tablespoons olive oil. Add the following spices to the oil and reduce to medium-low:

- Sea salt and pepper

- Turmeric

- Chili flakes (optional)

- Basil, oregano

- Cumin (seeds or powder)

- 1 clove crushed garlic

Sautee the above ingredients until they are all coated in oil and soften, which takes about 2-3 minutes. For the next step, add the following:

- 1 cup pureed tomatoes of tomato sauce

- Additional spices and/or herbs, if desired.

Stir the ingredients together, making sure they are all combined evenly, while keeping the cooking level on medium-low, then slightly increasing to medium, add any (all, some or none) of the following:

- Sliced green peppers

- Okra

- Bell peppers

- ½ cup ground beef, chicken or lamb (previously cooked until brown, with added spices)

- Sliced mushrooms

Add more ingredients not included in the list, as required, and continue to cook for another 5-7 minutes. Take two eggs and break them into the mixture, both in a central location of the skillet, so that they can absorb the surrounding flavors as they cook. Adding the two (or three) eggs should be done towards the end of preparing this dish so that they can cook without further stirring or mixing. Once the eggs are cooked and "settled," the dish is ready to serve right from the skillet.

There are many variations to this dish, which include the following toppings and ingredients for consideration:

- Add ½ cup of soft goat cheese or cream cheese to the tomato sauce to create a rose sauce

- Toppings can include dried or fresh parsley, dill, parmesan cheese or any variety of shredded cheese

- Bacon crumbles, as a topping or mixed into the tomato sauce

Casseroles

<u>Lasagne Options for Low Carb Diets</u>

During the colder seasons, casseroles and similar baking dishes are an excellent and easy way to prepare a meal. From lasagne to moussaka and other blends of vegetables and meats with various sauces and toppings, casseroles provide a hearty meal, and most often, a good portion of leftovers for the next day. A standard oven and a medium to large baking dish are the main requirements for assembling a good casserole meal.

Before you begin to prepare this dish, there are limitless recipes and options available, or you can simply invent your own casserole with the basic foundations of what's involved. This recipe provides a lot of options for changes and substitutes and can be easily adapted to a ketogenic or low carb diet. The first option is to choose the ingredients and "theme" of your casserole:

- Is the base of this dish tomato-based?

- Will cheese be an option as part of the ingredients and/or as a topping?

- Is this meal vegan or vegetarian?

If you choose to add meat to this dish, especially ground beef, pork, lamb and/or chicken, heat a skillet and cook until it is browned and seasoned, then set aside. The portion of meat prepared depends on how large your casserole will be, or simply how much meat you wish to include. This can be anywhere from ½ cup to 2 cups of cooked ground meat. Other ingredients to add may include diced onions, crushed garlic, chili flakes, salt, and pepper.

If you are making a lasagne dish, noodles are traditionally used in the layering process. For a low carb version of this recipe, thinly sliced eggplant, zucchini and/or cabbage leaves all make excellent substitutes. They can be added in between layers of cooked meat, shredded cheese and other vegetables, such as sliced carrots, basil leaves, peppers and/or mushrooms. If zucchini and/or eggplant are used in this recipe, they should be prepared ahead as follows:

- Slice the eggplant and/or zucchini thinly and lengthwise, then rinse in a colander

- Add a thin layer of salt to both sides of each slice and set aside for 20 minutes. This process effectively tenderizes the vegetable, making it easier to bake or cook

- Rinse the salt off the vegetable slices, and pat dry. They are now ready to use in making the lasagne

When preparing a layered casserole dish, including lasagne, always evenly coat the pan with olive oil, then add a thin layer of either tomato sauce or creamy cheese sauce (or a combination of both mixed together). This will keep the bottom of the pan from burning and prevent the ingredients from sticking. Add more layers, beginning with the thinly sliced zucchini and/or eggplant "noodles," or cabbage leaves. The addition or substitution of cabbage leaves will alter the taste of this casserole to a more cabbage-roll flavor, which may be a good option for some occasions. For the cabbage roll-lasagne variation, cheese can be omitted or added as a light topping.

After the initial layer, alternate between different vegetables, and/or meat with a sauce layer in between. In the end or top layer, sprinkle carefully and lightly with olive oil to avoid burning the casserole in the oven. Add a layer of spices, such as paprika, and pepper or sprinkle with shredded cheese or parmesan. Bake in a pre-heated oven for approximately 40 minutes on 350 degrees Fahrenheit. Depending on several factors, such as the number of ingredients, size of the dish, and types of ingredients used, baking may take more or less time. For this reason, check the oven frequently, in 5 to 6-minute intervals, beginning around 25 minutes and after. This will give you a good indication of how quickly the casserole of your choice will take when it is prepared again.

Cauliflower and Broccoli Cheese Bake

If you are looking for a simpler option that requires fewer ingredients and preparation, this option or a variation of this dish is an easy meal. It doesn't require any measurements or specifications, just the desired ingredients and a lot of cheese. If you're are vegan or prefer a plant-based option, there are a vegetable and soy-based vegan cheeses available in most grocery stores. For a creamier option, where the cheese component of this casserole is more rich and thicker, add cream cheese. For best results, melt the cream cheese in a microwave for 30-60 seconds, before adding to the other ingredients.

When you picture a macaroni and cheese bake, this casserole is basically the same idea, with the exception of replacing the noodles with the vegetable(s) of your choice. In combination with cheese flavors, broccoli and cauliflower are excellent options. They contain the right texture and compliment any type of cheese or combination of cheeses. This is also the case for vegan cheese, which tends to taste similar to dairy-based cheese. If it is essential to have vegan cheese that melts similarly to diary cheese, choose vegetable-based cheese options instead of soy-based, which doesn't melt as well.

To prepare this dish, grease a medium or large baking dish with olive oil and preheat the oven to 350 degrees. Prepare the broccoli and cauliflower by removing the stems and chopping the florets into small, 1-inch pieces. If only broccoli or cauliflower are available or only one of these options is preferred, double the amount of your choice. Once the vegetables are chopped equally in size, add to a large bowl and toss in at least 2 cups of shredded cheese, mixing thoroughly to coat. Add or sprinkle the equivalent of 2 teaspoons of olive oil into the bowl. Cheese options (dairy-based) to consider include:

- Shredded mozzarella, cheddar and/or Swiss cheese

- ½ cup of melted cream cheese (plain, unflavoured)

Other ingredients to consider adding to this recipe include:

- Bacon bits or crumble (optional) or the vegan version of the same

- Ground beef or the soy/vegan equivalent, fried or baked in a skillet

Pour the cheese-covered broccoli and/or cauliflower into the casserole dish, and top with paprika, pepper, shredded parmesan cheese and sprinkle with oil. Bake uncovered for 35 minutes. Keep an eye on the top of the casserole, to ensure it doesn't overcook. Additional cheese can be added to the top of this dish halfway through baking if preferred.

If neither cauliflower nor broccoli are available or preferred, brussels sprouts are a great option for baking, especially with parmesan cheese. They can be baked on their own in a medium baking dish, coated in oil and parmesan cheese, until they are slightly crispy on the outside. These make a great side dish or light meal.

Baking Vegetables: Keeping it Simple

There are some vegetables that are simply delicious on their own, with very little or nothing added, as they contain enough flavor on their own to carry a meal or side. The following vegetables are recommended, especially when they are in season and at their peak performance:

- Eggplant. Once prepared by soaking in salt for 20 minutes, eggplant slices can be baked on their own, sprinkled lightly with salt, or coated in parmesan cheese.

- Squash. Any variety of squash is an excellent meal on its own, due to its rich flavor and texture. To prepare, poke holes with a fork into the thick skin of the squash and bake for 10-15 minutes in 350 degrees. This will soften the vegetable and allow easier slicing to further bake for another 30-40 minutes until the inner flesh of the vegetable is tender. Coat with oil or butter before baking.

- Potatoes, yams, and sweet potatoes. All of these options take a while to bake, at least one hour, which makes them best to prepare when you have time to spare, or while preparing another dish. Smaller sizes of this vegetable bake faster. For good results, wrap in tin foil and poke with a fork to allow more even cooking.

- Radishes. This pungent tasting vegetable becomes much milder once it is roasted in the oven for 15-20 minutes. It can be cooked similarly to brussels sprouts, only without any added ingredients, with the exception of salt, butter or oil.

- Turnip or Rutabaga. This root vegetable becomes milder in flavor once it is baked. It is also used as a low carb alternative to potatoes and/or yams. These root vegetables can be shredded and fried similarly to potatoes or baked as well.

In general, root vegetables make great baking dishes, on their own or with other foods. Salt and olive oil or butter are the only ingredients needed to enhance the flavors of baked vegetables. They can also be baked in a small, covered baking dish with oil, salt and pepper and broth to add more flavor if desired. Miso paste can be added for more nutrients.

Salads

There are many options for salads, as there are ingredients to consider. Salads are a great opportunity to get the most out of leafy green vegetables while adding many other flavors to sweeten, spice or otherwise liven up the bitter flavors of arugula, spinach, and kale. Lettuce is another good option for a salad base, as it is neutral in flavor and offers a good source of iron and fiber. Kale, spinach, arugula and/or Swiss chard all offer a high level of nutrients and can be used either in combination or individually as a salad base. To build a salad, there are a few items to consider before preparation:

- Choose your base, preferably a leafy green: kale, cabbage, spinach, arugula, swiss chard, lettuce and/or others. Slice the green thin and combine in a large bowl

- Add to your greens: sprouts (pea sprouts, alfalfa, bean sprouts, etc.), other vegetables, such as carrots, broccoli, cucumber, edamame beans (shelled)

The dressing doesn't need to be fancy or loaded with ingredients. A simple balsamic dressing with oil and vinegar is healthy, low in carbohydrates and sugar, and very easy to make within a few minutes:

- Create a balsamic dressing by combining vinegar, olive oil (about 2-3 tablespoons each), and add flavor: freshly squeezed lime or lemon juice, dried rosemary leaves (crushed), mashed raspberries, or another option

Once the base ingredients are combined, and dressing is prepared, there are many toppings and other ingredients to consider adding to mix or on top of the salad:

- Baked chicken breast in basil leaves and olive oil (sliced into strips as a topping)

- Baked salmon

- Fried shrimp with butter and garlic

- Spicy tofu or tempeh cubes

- Shredded cheese (any variety)

- Nuts and seeds (pumpkin, flax or hemp seeds; almonds, walnuts, peanuts, cashews, hazelnuts, etc.). Nuts can be added raw, lightly salted or dry roasted on the stovetop, before adding as a topping to a salad

- Roasted root vegetables, such as baked squash or yams, sliced into cubes. Roasted or pickled beets are another option

- Boiled egg

There are countless ways to change and dress a salad, either for a regular meal or as a side dish. Salads that focus primarily on nutrient-rich and low carb ingredients are ideal before an intermittent fasting window or long-term fast. Salads are also a gentle way to effectively break a fast, as they provide a lot of healthy ingredients while not overwhelming the digestive system right after fasting.

Soups and Stews

A slow-cooked meal is a tasty option, though often overlooked in a busy society where meals are prepared quickly and without much thought. Soups and stews are best made over a period of hours, which can be done with a slow cooker while you're away at work, or overnight in preparation for the next day. Making large portions is advantageous for meal preparation over a week or several days in advance. Preparing a stew is as easy as choosing a broth or soup base, herbs, and spices, as well as the ingredients. Beef stew is an exceptional way to add a significant source of iron, protein, and calcium to a meal, along with other vegetables and spices to add fiber and vitamins, including antioxidants. Meat can be substituted for tempeh or tofu, and a vegetable soup base or broth can be flavored further with miso or soy sauce.

The broth or soup base should be as natural as possible, either through careful selection at a grocery store or by preparing the broth homemade with soup bones and vegetable rinds. The broth or base should be plain, and all spices and flavors added, such as bay leaves, sea salt, pepper, basil and other options as desired. Turmeric and paprika make great options as well.

Stewing beef should be added first to the broth, as it takes the longest to cook. Other vegetables and ingredients can be added later, once the beef is cooked and becomes tender:

- Celery (sliced in small, bite-sized pieces)

- Carrots, sliced

- Potatoes cut into cubes (or turnips, for a low carb option)

- Asparagus

- Spinach

- Onion (minced)

- Garlic cloves (crushed)

- Chili flakes and/or cayenne pepper

Soy sauce can be added in small amounts to boost the flavor of the stew. Salt and pepper are also good options to enhance the beef flavor. Stewing this dish can be easily done over a period of 6-8 hours on low heat. The recommended amount of broth or soup base is eight cups or more, to ensure all of the ingredients are covered and submerged. Adding more ingredients and using a larger cooking pot would require more broth.

Soup Options

Creamy soups are often coconut milk or dairy milk-based and can add another level of taste to a simple soup. Curried soups are usually prepared with a coconut milk base, with spices including curry powder, added. Preparing a curry soup is as simple as adding coconut milk and curry spices to a vegetable or meat-based broth or soup base, then adding the ingredients. To make a soup creamy, simply add cream to the broth, along with the various vegetables. Once the ingredients are cooked, remove from the heat and blend in a food processor, then reheat to serve.

If you are looking to add healthy, natural sources of carbs for energy to a soup, consider lentils, chickpeas, kidney beans, and black beans as options, as well as barley and quinoa as healthy grain options that also provide a high nutrient count. Avoid refined pasta and rice as much as possible and add as many whole food options. Ideal vegetables to blend for creamy or thickening soups include pumpkin (in pureed form), squash and carrots. Broccoli, potato, and cauliflower are options that may be added together or separately to make a hearty soup.

Chili Options

Like stews, chilis are a great way to provide a filling meal, while staying warm during colder months. Chili is traditionally made with beans, though this option can be omitted to adjust for a lower carb version. Tomato paste and sauce are the first ingredients to begin with, which can be made at home or store-bought. Stewing tomatoes with pureed sauce and paste can be further enhanced with sliced tomatoes, so that they can be stewed to absorb the flavors, in combination with cayenne, chili flakes, black pepper, and paprika. Ground beef or a vegetarian meat substitute is added to stir with the tomato sauce, followed by the following ingredients:

- Sliced green peppers and/or bell peppers

- Diced jalapeno peppers (sliced thinly)

- Okra

- Zucchini (sliced)

- Mushrooms

- Spinach

- Onions (diced)

- Garlic (crushed)

Chili is stewed slowly, over a period of a few hours, to get the most flavor out of all ingredients combined. The longer the duration, the stronger the flavor. If a large enough stew is prepared, the chili can last for several days as a main meal or in combination with other foods. It makes a great dinner or small portion size with eggs in the morning. As a light meal, it can be served in a bowl topped with shredded cheese or with salad.

Smoothies

One of the best ways to get nutrients quickly and efficiently is with a smoothie or milkshake. If you have any variety of milk (dairy or non-dairy), various fruits and some ice in the freezer, you already have most, if not all the basic ingredients to make a smoothie. In addition to the basics, there are other options to add for boost the protein and nutrient levels in your smoothie, including:

- Any variety of nut butter, such as peanut, almond, hazelnut or sesame butter. Just one tablespoon can provide a substantial amount of protein in your smoothie

- Most smoothies add a banana for its thickening effect and the added flavor. Avocados make a great low carb alternative to bananas and can be added to almost any combination of fruits. On their own, avocados are a great milkshake combined with coconut, almond or dairy milk as a base.

- Hemp seeds, flax seeds, and plant-based proteins: these can be either crushed into a powder or small granules, like hemp or flax or bought as a fine powder in most bulk stores. The types of plant-based proteins are limitless and include everything from soy, pumpkin, hemp and chia seed varieties. Chia seeds on their own make another great addition, due to their high calcium and fiber.

- MCT oil or coconut oil. This is a beneficial way to add more healthy fats to your diet, especially if you adhere to a strict ketogenic diet. MCT oil is not as common in grocery stores as coconut oil, though it can be ordered online or purchased in most natural food stores.

- Kale, spinach and other leafy greens can make an excellent addition to a fruit-based smoothie. Their strong, bitter flavor is offset by the natural sweetness of watermelon, cantaloupe, and other melon juices, or mango and orange juice. If you choose to use juice as a base instead of milk, avoid the packaged variety and try making your own homemade juice with a juicer, blender or by simply hand-squeezing citrus fruits. Watermelon is a good choice, due to how quickly it can be blended in a food processor and added to a smoothie. Mangoes and citrus fruits combined also make a great option as a base for a green smoothie

- Green tea, more specifically matcha, is usually available in powder form and makes a great energy boost to any smoothie. There is a high level of antioxidants in green tea that rival many fresh fruits and vegetables. If fresh or frozen fruits are limited, green tea powder is a good substitute with coconut milk and either avocado or banana.

New supplements, "boosters" and various nutrient enhancements are becoming more readily available, with more plant-based and low carb options that include high levels of vitamins, proteins, and ingredients not always available in fresh fruits and vegetables. These are especially beneficial for long-term shelf life and increasing the meal replacement value of a smoothie, which can be a great option for breakfast or in between meals as a snack. The following ingredient combinations are suggestions for different flavors, and can be modified or changed according to personal preference:

<u>Low Carb Smoothie Options:</u>

- Avocado (ripe), coconut milk, matcha green tea powder and low carb sweetener (monk fruit or stevia)

- Berries, almond milk (or dairy, coconut milk) with tahini (sesame butter)

- Dark cocoa (unsweetened) with almond milk, peanut or hazelnut butter

- Pumpkin puree, cinnamon and almond milk with hemp seeds or protein powder

Moderate Carb/High Energy Options for Workouts:

- Bananas, avocado, coconut or almond milk, and low carb sweetener

- Berries, bananas, milk, and hemp protein

- Mangoes, coconut milk, cardamom powder and low carb sweetener (peaches can also be used as a substitute)

Juice-Based Smoothies:

- Orange juice, mangoes, bananas, and pumpkin protein powder

- Watermelon (or cantaloupe, honeydew) with pineapple, mango and/or peaches. Add lime or lime and leafy greens, such as kale, mint or spinach leaves

Another option to consider adding to a smoothie for flavor, nutrients, and thickening the texture is yogurt or kefir. Both options contain bacterial cultures beneficial for gut health and are best used in a plain, unsweetened form. Kefir contains a higher level of probiotics and tends to be thinner than regular yogurt, which makes it an ideal option for smoothies. Yogurt, while it is thicker, can be added to almond or coconut milk. Yogurt and kefir-based smoothies can be prepared similarly to milk and non-dairy milk-based varieties.

Fermented Foods

One of the healthiest types of foods on the planet is fermented vegetables, dairy, and soy. The most familiar varieties are yogurt and kefir for dairy, tempeh, and miso for soy and kimchi and sauerkraut for vegetables. All fermented foods have a direct impact on improving gut health, which is essential in digesting and properly utilizing all of the nutrients we receive from the foods we eat. Fermented foods are also very convenient and often available in most grocery stores or delis. They have been associated with the prevention of certain cancers, and digestive diseases, and promote weight loss while supporting the metabolism. The strong level of nutrients in kimchi and sauerkraut make them ideal side dishes, which is usually how they are served, either on the side of a dish or in a small bowl. These foods are also very filling in small doses and can be used sparingly with stews and stir fry meals.

Sauerkraut, kimchi, and yogurt can be made at home by following a recipe or bought already prepared for convenience. Fermented soy, such as miso and tempeh, go through a longer process. In order to produce miso, the fermentation process can take weeks, months, and for some varieties, years to make. The longer the duration of fermenting, the stronger the taste and flavor. Miso is beneficial in small amounts in soups, dips and as an added ingredient to stews and sautés. Fermented foods have a long shelf life and once opened, can be refrigerated for at least one week or more.

All of the above foods, recipes, suggestions, and ideas can build a solid start to a healthy diet that can support intermittent fasting and prepare the body for longer-term fasting goals. Overall, most people don't always take into consideration the quality of foods they eat when they consider fasting as an option, and instead, focus on the fasting process itself. While this is important, the foods we eat around those fasting windows is equally vital to ensuring we have all the nutrients we require to sustain our bodies through a fast, and as we move towards a state of autophagy.

Chia Seed Puddings

A simple yet very effective way to increase the nutrient content of your meal is by adding chia seeds. They contain a significant source of plant-based protein, calcium, vitamins, fiber, and antioxidants. Chia seeds are great for creating puddings from milk, as they expand in liquid and create a thick, custard-like texture. Their taste adapts to the ingredients combined with them, and they are excellent for vegan diets that are also low carb or ketogenic. In its simple form, chia seed pudding can be prepared as follows:

- 2 cups milk (dairy, coconut or almond milk)

- ½ cup full-fat cream (dairy or coconut cream)

- 2-3 teaspoons low carb sweetener (monk fruit, stevia or a blend)

- 1 teaspoon vanilla extract

Combine all of the ingredients in a medium to large bowl and mix evenly, to ensure all chia seeds are distributed throughout the milk. Add cinnamon and more sweetener as needed. Refrigerate for at least two hours to thicken the pudding and serve. Preparing this dish and refrigerating overnight is a good option for enjoying immediately in the morning, with no further preparation time needed. There are many other flavors and options to consider when preparing this pudding by adding the following:

- Sprinkle the top of the pudding with cinnamon or cardamom just prior to serving

- Combine fresh fruits, such as berries and currents, to enhance the flavor of the pudding. These can be added during the mixing of the ingredients, or later, once the pudding has formed.

- Add dark cocoa or chocolate (unsweetened) to the pudding, along with chocolate flakes or shavings as a topping or ingredient.

- Coconut flakes, slivered almonds, crushed pecans, walnuts or pistachios are all great options to add flavor to the pudding

- Hemp hearts and flax seeds can enhance the healthy fats and protein content of the pudding.

Chia seed pudding offers a lot of options to mix and match various flavors and experiment with your own tastes. The best advantage of this dish is its dessert-like quality, which is also very nutritious and fitting as a full meal in itself. It can serve as a meal replacement at any time of day.

How Does Intermittent Fasting Combine with a Low Carb Diet?

Implementing both a fasting schedule with dietary changes is an involving task, though it provides a lot of options on planning and scheduling. The following sample plans indicate how to use various diet options in conjunction with intermittent fasting plans, starting from 12:12 (twelve hours fasting, twelve hours eating) as a starting point:

12:12 Intermittent Fasting Sample: Plan A

This plan begins the beginner level of fasting for 12 hours at an early 6 am start.

12:12 sample daily plan (any weekday or weekend)	Fasting/eating schedule from 6 am to 6 pm
6 am	Begin eating window. Coffee or tea, water. Scrambled eggs or tofu with fresh fruit or avocado
12 pm – 1 pm	Lunch break: salad with baked salmon and a side of kimchi
3 pm	Snack (optional). Yogurt with fruit, or a smoothie
5 pm – 6 pm	Dinner: baked casserole or stew with a side salad Coffee or tea
6 pm until 6 am the following day	Fasting begins immediately after dinner and lasts for 12 hours until the following

	day at 6 am when breakfast is served.

12:12 Intermittent Fasting Sample: Plan B

This version or option for the 12-hour fasting plan begins slightly later in the morning, at 8am. This can be further shifted to begin at 9, or 10 am, though keep in mind the duration of the eating window ends exactly 12 hours later, into the late evening:

12:12 sample daily plan (any weekday or weekend)	Fasting/eating schedule from 8 am to 8 pm
8 am	Begin eating window. Coffee or tea, water. Scrambled eggs or tofu with fresh fruit or avocado
1 pm – 2 pm	Lunch break: salad with baked salmon and a side of kimchi
4 pm	Snack (optional). Yogurt with fruit, or a smoothie
6 pm – 8 pm	Dinner: baked casserole or stew with a side salad Coffee or tea
8 pm until 8 am the following day	Fasting begins immediately after dinner and lasts for 12 hours until the following

	day at 6 am when breakfast is served.

16:8 Intermittent Fasting Sample: Plan A

After a few weeks of 12:12, moving into a longer fasting phase is recommended to adjust your body to a longer period of abstaining from food and drink. The following sample uses the same food options as 12:12 to illustrate how they would be adjusted to accommodate a change in hours. The significant change is in the increase of 12 to 16 hours of fasting while maintaining a similar eating schedule:

16:8 sample daily plan (any weekday or weekend)	Fasting/eating schedule from 6 am to 2 pm
6 am	Begin eating window. Coffee or tea, water. Scrambled eggs or tofu with fresh fruit or avocado.
11 am – 12 pm	Lunch break: salad with baked salmon and a side of kimchi. A mid-morning snack is also an option, such as yogurt with chia seeds and fruits or a smoothie.
1 pm - 2 pm	Light lunch or mid-afternoon snack. The two eating options suggested between 11

	am – 12 pm and 1 – 2 pm can be interchangeable, depending on your schedule and preference.
2 pm – 6 am the next morning	Fasting begins at 2 pm and lasts until the next day at 6 am. Dinner is skipped completely. Bone broth and/or tea are options during the fasting period.

<u>16:8 Intermittent Fasting Sample: Plan B</u>

The following sample starts at a later time to show how traditional meals can be further adjusted within the 8-hour range. In plan A, the dinner is skipped completely, with a focus on breakfast and lunch, with an option for a mid-morning or mid-afternoon snack. In this schedule, the eating window begins later, after breakfast:

16:8 sample daily plan (any weekday or weekend)	**Fasting/eating schedule from 10 am to 6 pm**
10 am	Begin eating window. Smoothie with fruit and protein or yogurt, chia seeds and fresh fruits. Prior to 10 am, during a fasting window, bone broth, coffee, and tea are options.
1 pm – 2 pm	Lunch break: salad with baked salmon and

	a side of kimchi. This lunch period can be shifted to a later start time, between 2-3 pm.
5 pm – 6 pm	Dinner options include a casserole, stir fry or skillet meal or baked vegetables with a choice of protein.
6 pm – 10 am the next morning	Fasting begins at 6 pm and lasts until the next day at 10 am. Breakfast is either skipped the next morning completely or moved to a later time, starting 10 am or later. Bone broth and/or tea are options during the fasting period.

16:8 Intermittent Fasting Sample: Plan C:

Applying the same 8-hour fasting window as in plans A and B for the 16:8 fasting schedule, the following option is ideal for late shift work or a later start in the day:

16:8 sample daily plan (any weekday or weekend)	Fasting/eating schedule from 1 pm to 9 pm
1 pm	Begin the eating window and break your fast with a light salad, followed by a

	nutritious lunch: stir fry, lasagne, soup or stew. Sushi with a side of edamame beans and/or kimchi.
5 pm – 7 pm	Dinner can be served at this time. This may include a skillet, soup, stew or chili. No further meals are required following the dinner, or a light snack can be added just prior to beginning the fasting window.
8 pm – 9 pm	A light snack is optional and may include fresh fruits, black olives with guacamole and/or cheese or miso soup with tofu and seaweed.
9 pm – 1 pm the next day	Fasting begins at 9 pm and lasts until the next day at 1 pm. Breakfast is skipped completely, and a light snack or meal can be enjoyed as lunch. Bone broth and/or tea are options during the fasting period.

The next step in the progression to longer fasting intervals is a slight increase from 16 to 18 hours of fasting. While this may not seem like a significant change, the two-hour difference can signify the start of autophagy, which can begin as early as 18 hours into a fasting window. For most people, this process doesn't begin until 24 hours, though there is a chance that some of the benefits could start as early as 18 hours, which makes this step all the more crucial in adapting to this diet.

<u>18:6 Intermittent Fasting Sample: Plan A:</u>

The 18:6 intermittent fasting schedule allows for a 6-hour window for eating, which represents one-quarter of a full 24-hour day. To get the most out of this plan, center your eating plan around two meals instead of three, and include as many nutrients as possible. The sample meals below are simply guidelines, which can be replaced with other options:

18:6 sample daily plan (any weekday or weekend)	Fasting/eating schedule from 7 am to 1 pm
7 am	Begin the eating window with a hearty breakfast, which may include eggs, tofu, fresh herbs, skillet-fried vegetables with a side of bacon or ham and a small bowl of fruit. This meal essentially breaks the fast from the night before, which lasts from 1 pm to 7 am.
10:30 am – 11 am	Lunch can be served at an earlier time, between 10:30 and 1 pm, or this small timeframe can be a suitable option for a mid-morning snack, followed by lunch or larger meal between 12 pm – 1 pm.
12 pm – 1 pm	This is the last meal prior to beginning the

	fasting window. Add as many nutrients and proteins as possible. If you plan to eat a spicy meal, add a small cup of yogurt to aid in digestion. This is a good option for any dish, particularly where foods can be challenging or slow to digest, such as certain spices and meats.
1 pm – 7 am the next morning	Fasting begins at 1 pm and lasts until the next day at 7 am. Dinner is skipped completely. Bone broth and/or tea are options during the fasting period.

18:6 Intermittent Fasting Sample: Plan B:

The second 18:6 option or plan starts the eating window later in the morning, omitting breakfast completely and focusing on lunch and an early dinner. To get the most out of this plan, center your eating around the lunch hour, adding an optional light snack before and/or after and include as many nutrients as possible. The sample meals below are simply guidelines, which can be replaced with other options:

18:6 sample daily plan (any weekday	Fasting/eating schedule from 11 am to 5 pm

or weekend)	
11 am	Begin the eating window with a light mid-morning snack, such as avocado, one or two boiled eggs, and miso soup. A chia seed pudding and/or yogurt with fruits are good options. This meal essentially breaks the fast from the night before, which lasts from 5 pm to 11 am.
1 pm – 2 pm	Lunch can be served at an earlier time, between 1 pm and 2 pm, followed by dinner or a larger meal between 4 pm – 5 pm.
4 pm – 5 pm	This is the last meal prior to beginning the fasting window. Add as many nutrients and proteins as possible. If you plan to eat a spicy meal, add a small cup of yogurt to aid in digestion. This is a good option for any dish, particularly where foods can be challenging or slow to digest, such as certain spices and meats.
5 pm – 11 am the next morning	Fasting begins at 5 pm and lasts until the next day at 11 am. Breakfast is skipped completely. Bone broth and/or tea are options during the fasting period.

The final suggested plan starts at lunch and allows for more flexibility between the lunch and dinner meals while skipping breakfast entirely. For added nutrients in the morning, enjoy a cup of bone broth and coffee. Drink plenty of water during the fasting hours.

18:6 Intermittent Fasting Sample: Plan C:

18:6 sample daily plan (any weekday or weekend)	Fasting/eating schedule from 1 pm to 7 pm
1 pm	Begin the eating window with a light salad or snack, followed by a lunch that contains a lot of nutrients. This meal essentially breaks the fast from the night before, which lasts from 7 pm to 1 pm
4 pm – 5 pm	Dinner can be served at an earlier time, preferably between 4 pm – 5 pm. A light snack may also be added around 3 pm as an appetizer, or as a more substantial snack or dessert after this meal.
6 pm – 7 pm	This is the last meal prior to beginning the fasting window. Even a small portion

	snack or light meal can contain a lot of nutrients. If you plan to eat a spicy meal, add a small cup of yogurt to aid in digestion. This is a good option for any dish, particularly where foods can be challenging or slow to digest, such as certain spices and meats.
7 pm – 1 pm the next day	Fasting begins at 7 pm and lasts until the next day at 1 pm Breakfast is skipped completely. Bone broth and/or tea are options during the fasting period.

The next phase in intermittent fasting is moving from 18 hours to 20 hours, bringing the "sweet spot" or peak of autophagy even closer. 20 hours marks an important milestone, as it is usually the last stop before trying a full day 24-hour fast. The 20:4 method focuses mostly on one meal or series of healthy foods within a 4-hour window of opportunity:

20:4 Intermittent Fasting Sample: Plan A

20:4 sample daily plan (any weekday or weekend)	Fasting/eating schedule from 8 am to 12 pm

8 am to 12 pm	This is a four-hour fasting window that can begin with either a light start, such as a bowl of fresh fruit and cream, or yogurt, followed by an egg dish loaded with as many nutrients and vitamins as possible. If you start work or become busy within this eating window, be sure to add another small meal or snack within the 11 am to 12 pm or final hour of the window, just prior to beginning the fast.
12 pm – 8 am	Fasting begins at 12 pm, following a light lunch or healthy snack, and lasts until 8 am the next morning. Drink plenty of water, and supplement with bone broth or tea if needed. Coffee can also be added during this time. To increase the chances of achieving autophagy during a 20-hour fast, try dry fasting by omitting all fluids during the fasting window. This will allow your body to use up its resources faster.

Using the same meal ideas in the first plan, the 4-hour window can be moved to a later time in the day, to focus around lunch hour. This is particularly useful is you have a flexible schedule that will accommodate a snack during a break and lunch. Breakfast and dinner meals are omitted completely:

<u>20:4 Intermittent Fasting Sample: Plan B</u>

20:4 sample daily plan (any weekday or weekend)	Fasting/eating schedule from 11 am to 3 pm
11 am to 3 pm	This is a four-hour fasting window that can begin with either a light start, such as a bowl of fresh fruit and cream, or yogurt, followed by an egg dish loaded with as many nutrients and vitamins as possible. This meal can either serve as a late breakfast or early lunch. If you start work or become busy within this eating window, be sure to add another small meal or snack within the 2 pm to 3 pm or final hour of the window, just prior to beginning the fast.
3 pm – 11 am	Fasting begins at 3 pm, following a light lunch or healthy snack, and lasts until 8 am the next morning. Drink plenty of water, and supplement with bone broth or

	tea if needed. Coffee can also be added during this time. To increase the chances of achieving autophagy during a 20-hour fast, try dry fasting by omitting all fluids during the fasting window. This will allow your body to use up its resources faster.

The following two samples plans C and D, illustrate the increased flexibility of a reduced eating window, and the availability to move the preferred mealtimes within those hours. As restrictive as the time frame may appear, the plan itself allows for variances in when the hours are scheduled and can provide opportunities to learn and discover which time of the day works best for eating versus fasting:

<u>20:4 Intermittent Fasting Sample: Plan C</u>

20:4 sample daily plan (any weekday or weekend)	Fasting/eating schedule from 6 am to 10 am
6 am to 10 am	This is a four-hour fasting window that can begin with either a light start, such as a bowl of fresh fruit and cream, or yogurt,

	followed by an egg dish loaded with as many nutrients and vitamins as possible. If you start work or become busy within this eating window, be sure to add another small meal or snack within the 9 am, and 10 am or final hour of the window, just prior to beginning the fast. This specific plan works within the breakfast hours of the day, which can have the benefit of spreading out two meals or light snacking throughout this time frame until fasting begins at 10 am.
10 am – 6 am	Fasting begins at 10 am, following a light lunch or healthy snack, and lasts until 6 am the next morning. Drink plenty of water, and supplement with bone broth or tea if needed. Coffee can also be added during this time. Lunch and dinner are skipped in favor of maximizing the nutrients and good food choices within the early hours of the day. To increase the chances of achieving autophagy during a 20-hour fast, try dry fasting by omitting all fluids during the

	fasting window. This will allow your body to use up its resources faster.

20:4 Intermittent Fasting Sample: Plan D

20:4 sample daily plan (any weekday or weekend)	Fasting/eating schedule from 4 pm to 8 pm
4 pm to 8 pm	This is a four-hour fasting window that can begin with a salad or soup, followed by a casserole, skillet meal, or similar dish. As the evening progresses, there is the option for a light snack, such as yogurt, fresh fruit, or an egg or avocado, prior to beginning the fasting window at 8 pm. If you have a tendency to become hungry in the morning, be sure to include a lot of nutritious, slow-digesting foods. Include fermented food options within the 4-hour window, and this will help the next morning. This specific plan works around the dinner hour, which can have the benefit of

	spreading out two meals or light snacking throughout this time frame until fasting begins at 8 pm.
8 pm to 4 pm the next day	Fasting begins at 8 pm. Drink plenty of water, and supplement with bone broth or tea if needed. Coffee can also be added during this time. Breakfast and lunch are skipped in favor of maximizing the nutrients and good food choices within the evening hours of the day. To increase the chances of achieving autophagy during a 20-hour fast, try dry fasting by omitting all fluids during the fasting window. This will allow your body to use up its resources faster.

The 24-hour fasting method is your ideal goal to reach autophagy and moving through all of the shorter intermittent fasting plans will place you in a position for success. As you approach this as your next option, keep the following in mind as you prepare to begin a full day fast:

- Start your first 24-hour fast with plenty of water and acceptable liquids. Avoid dry fasting unless you have tried shorter fasting periods with no fluids or have completed a regular full-day fast several times successfully.

- Prior to ending your eating window, eat a hearty, nutritious meal within the last hour before you begin your fast. This will give your body a good foundation for using high-quality nutrients right up until the process of autophagy begins

- Exercise during the early part of your fast, to increase the metabolic rate, which can move you into autophagy faster as well.

- Bone broth is a good option to keep the nutrient level high during your fast, though it may have the effect of slowing down progression towards autophagy. If you are able to avoid most fluids, and only use water during the fast, this is an ideal situation. Water fasting ensures that you don't lose any hydration during the fasting process.

- Take time to meditate and slowly ease yourself into the fasting window. Don't view this process as a shift from one extreme to another, but rather as a transition from using food to taking a break during the fasting window. Your body will adjust, even if the initial experiences are challenging and with feelings of hunger. These symptoms will pass over time and make your body stronger and more resilient.

- Keep your schedule the same, if possible, and make sure you are getting enough hours of sleep. If you are content with the level of sleep and activities in your life currently, avoid making any radical or significant changes, as this will only cause more stress during the intermittent fasting process. The idea is to make this process as easy and gentle as possible.

As with longer fasting periods, which last over 24 hours, the same principles apply to the preparation and getting used to the new benefits and long-term opportunities that fasting and autophagy have to offer.

Chapter 7: Different Goals and Reasons for Using Autophagy and Low Carb Eating in Life

Disease Prevention

Autophagy is one of the best defenses against disease prevention because it functions so effectively at the cellular level. In maximizing the quality production of healthy cells, the chances of mutated and damaged cell production, often resulting from free radicals and other toxins in the body, are minimized, because of the food we eat and the opportunity we give our bodies to reuse the cell and tissue waste that would otherwise cause more problems in our bodies, if left as is.

Examples of the types of diseases and conditions that can be prevented or treated during autophagy include lowering cholesterol and maintaining healthy blood pressure level, preventing Alzheimer's and inflammation in the brain and body, and improving the function of the intestines and digestive system.

Cognitive Function and Brain Health

The nature of autophagy is to improve the quality and function of our body through cellular regeneration. This includes improving the way our brain functions, including memory, cognitive abilities, and focus. In improving how our brain works, memory loss and related diseases can be prevented and/or their progress slowed down to a manageable level.

Weight Loss

One of the most popular reasons to strive for ketosis and autophagy is the benefits of weight loss. Burning fat for fuel instead of glucose is a direct way of losing weight while increasing energy levels and other advantages that follow. There are many case studies that indicate how easily the body can move into a fat-adapted state and continuously burn for weeks or months at a time, while ketosis is regularly achieved.

Treatment of disease and disorders

While autophagy continues to be researched and studied to document its effects, some of the key findings to date include the prevention and treatment of some common diseases. One of the fascinating aspects of this process is the ability to suppress and reverse certain cancerous growths, including tumors. While the cellular regeneration process breaks down old cell waste for repairing damaged tissue and building new cells, it may also inhibit cancerous or mutated cell growth, either stopping or slowing the progression in its tracks. The very nature of autophagy is to promote and strengthen the growth of new cells, so that they perform and function better than before, preventing the start of many diseases of conditions.

The rebuilding and strengthening process at a cellular level would support an improved defense against certain heart conditions and their progression. Certain autoimmune and chronic conditions, such as arthritis, fibromyalgia, as well as inflammation and diseases that impact digestion may also improve over time due to autophagy.

Strengthening the Immune System

Stronger, newer cells will build a solid foundation for an immune system that functions well and can fight off viruses and disease more effectively. While our dietary habits play a key role in building and maintaining and supporting a powerful immune system, the recycling effect of old cells to produce more efficient cellular material can impact every aspect of the way our body functions, from prevention to treatment of mild to serious conditions. If your health is generally good and there are no known conditions, autophagy will continue to keep your immunity level at a high functioning rate, even as we age.

Anti-aging: The Ultimate Benefit of Autophagy

As popular as weight loss is for diet and fasting, as well as the benefits of treating disease, one major fascination with the science of autophagy is its ability to slow down, and to some degree, possibly reverse the aging process. As cells regenerate in smaller numbers as we age, their quality becomes increasingly more important. Some studies indicate that these newer cells have a restorative effect on our bodies, and organs, resulting in improved function. Visually, the skin may become firmer or retain more of its elasticity, due to improved performance of skin cells. In some cases where skin becomes loose, due to rapid weight loss and/or aging, there have been some improvements in reversing and improving this as well. Combining the efforts of a ketogenic diet and the benefits of autophagy will greatly increase the anti-aging effects both have on the body, both inside and out.

Chapter 8: Frequently Asked Questions, Tips, and Encouragement for Long-Term Success and Benefits of the Autophagy Diet

The autophagy diet or pathways to achieving a state of autophagy can be challenging and rewarding at the same time. In order to better understand and tackle some common issues and concerns associated with the benefits and struggles of shifting into a low carb diet and intermittent fasting, to produce results, the following frequently asked questions may prove helpful:

Q: How do I know when I reach autophagy?

A: The only way to detect the onset of autophagy is to verify the body's production of autophagosomes. While this is done in a lab for research purposes, it's not detectable through a home test kit. There are ways to detect if you are close to achieving this goal by testing for the production of ketones during a state of ketosis. Test strip kits can be purchased at many pharmacies over the counter and are usually accurate. Once you reach a state of ketosis, this means your body is burning fat and your cells will soon, if not already, search for materials for rebuilding. At this stage, you are close to reaching autophagy. Implementing a regular schedule of intermittent fasting, of at least 18 hours or more, in combination with low carb or ketogenic eating, is the best way to reach autophagy quickly.

Q: How often do I need to fast for autophagy to work?

A: This is an individual choice, depending on how often you wish to reach a state of autophagy, and will determine how often you fast. For example, fasting twice a week for 24-hours will help you reach this goal at least twice within the week. Longer fasts will take you to this goal as well and prolong the effects until you begin to eat again. Autophagy is not a process that occurs quickly, though once it is achieved, the benefits begin immediately. How often you choose to strive for this state is based on personal goals. Once or twice a week is a good start to see the results within a month.

Q: What is the best time frame for fasting to reach autophagy?

A: A 24-hour fast is an ideal goal for reaching the standard beginning of autophagy. Shorter fasting windows are a means to prepare and work towards this goal. If you choose to try dry fasting, your autophagy goal could be reached a bit sooner, between 18-24 hours, though using the 24-hour mark as a goal is based primarily on the findings that support a major increase in the production of autophagosomes at this stage. Expanding the fasting window to beyond the 24-hour window will continue the benefits of autophagy, once it is reached, though the benefits begin to plateau or lessen over time. In general, the 24-hour goal is the best option.

Q: What foods should I avoid within the eating window during intermittent fasting?

A: Low carb and ketogenic foods are strongly recommended, as they support the benefits of ketosis and autophagy, so eating anything outside of these options should be avoided unless you choose to add carbohydrates for energy at certain intervals. In general, avoid all refined and processed foods. This includes eliminating trans fats and chemically flavored foods that provide no nutritional benefit. While the occasional high carb treat isn't going to ruin a dietary plan, it can be habit-forming and addictive, especially if old eating habits included a lot of processed foods. Becoming accustomed to whole natural foods makes decisions a lot easier during eating windows.

Q: Can I exercise during a fast?

A: Yes. Exercise is good during a fast, as it speeds up towards autophagy, though if you feel faint or otherwise not comfortable engaging in high impact exercise, slow down. Yoga, stretching, and walking are all suitable ways to improve your fitness level while supporting your body's processes during a fast.

Tips for Achieving Autophagy Success

As long as you persevere and continue to improve, and work through the challenges of both ketogenic eating and intermittent fasting, there is no failure, only success. If you experience a setback, remember that it is a learning process. Making significant changes to the way you eat and live is not a simple procedure that can happen in one day. It is a lifestyle adjustment that can take weeks, months, and longer to fully implement, though the advantages are enormous and will sustain your health in the long-term. Keep in mind the following tips for achieving your goal towards autophagy:

- Document your progress and keep a list of foods that work and don't fit within your plan. This will keep your grocery shopping easy.

- Give yourself time. If you break your fast early during the first, second, or more times, it's completely acceptable. Our bodies are good at adapting, but it takes longer for some of us than others.

- Allow yourself a break once in a while. Intermittent fasting doesn't have to be constant or even consistent if it doesn't always fit into your goals. You can take a break for days or a week at a time to enjoy a vacation or time away and jump into it at a later date.

Once you become used to the routine of low carb meals and intermittent fasting, taking a break now and again, as well as increasing your efforts will become easier and more enjoyable, especially once you begin to see the results of your effort. Achieving autophagy is a life-long process that can lead to a longer, healthier life for many people, and also build confidence and strength in your mind and body for a better quality of life.